MRI Made Easy

Govind B Chavhan
MD DNB
Associate Radiologist
Jankharia Imaging
Mumbai

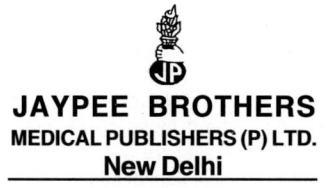

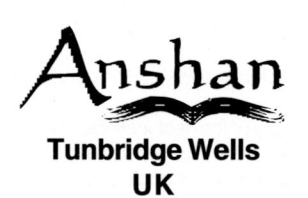

JAYPEE BROTHERS
MEDICAL PUBLISHERS (P) LTD.
New Delhi

Anshan
Tunbridge Wells
UK

First published in the UK by

Anshan Ltd
in 2007
6 Newlands Road
Tunbridge Wells
Kent TN4 9AT, UK

Tel: +44 (0)1892 557767
Fax: +44 (0)1892 530358
E-mail: info@anshan.co.uk
www.anshan.co.uk

Copyright © 2007 by (author)
Reprint 2010

The right of (author) to be identified as the author of this work has been asserted in accordance with the Copyright, Designs and Patents act 1988.

ISBN 10 1-905740-61-1
ISBN 13 978-1-905740-61-1

British Library Cataloguing in Publication Data
A catalogue record for this book is available from the British Library

All rights reserved. No part of this publication may be reproduced, stored in a retrieval system, or transmitted in any form or by any means, electronic, mechanical, photocopying, recording and/or otherwise without the prior written permission of the publishers. This book may not be lent, resold, hired out or otherwise disposed of by way of trade in any form, binding or cover other than that in which it is published, without the prior consent of the publishers.

Printed in India by Rajkamal Electric Press, Kundli, Haryana.

Many of the designations used by manufacturers and sellers to distinguish their products are claimed as trademarks. Where those designations appear in this book and where the publisher was aware of a trademark claim, the designations have been printed in initial capital letters.

To
Ravi Sir (Prof Ravi Ramakantan)
the teacher par excellence
unchallengeable Radiologist
'Niswarth Karmayogi' relentlessly working towards
the benefit of thousands of poor patients
the great igniter of minds
this is for you

Preface

Radiology is the fastest advancing branch of medical sciences. It is moving from evaluation of anatomy to physiology, structural to functional, morphological to tissue diagnosis and biochemical information. MR takes the lead in this rapid march of advancement of radiology. No other modality has developed so much as MR in last 20 years. MR has emerged as strong modality, which gives final answer in many conditions in all body systems.

This short introductory book is the superficial overview of the subject explaining the basic fundamentals. This work is done keeping in mind needs of the person beginning to learn MR, specially radiology residents. In attempt to simplify the subject, many complex things have purposely been omitted. This book is by no means complete source of the subject. This should serve as an appetizer for further reading of this interesting subject.

This book is divided into two sections. First section deals with basic principles, instrumentation of MR system, sequences and artifacts. Also discussed are few basic principles of MR interpretations. Section two has some advances and higher applications of MR. Following are few things to remember while reading this book:

- Start reading from the first chapter and go in sequence for better understanding.

- Protons, nuclei and spins are used synonymously; so do not get confused by them. They are one and the same.
- For quick reference to the sequence, list of the common sequences with their long forms is given in the beginning.

Govind B Chavhan

Acknowledgements

I am fortunate enough to work under idols like Dr. Bhavin Jankharia and Dr. Meher Ursekar. Their immense knowledge and vast experience, to remain up-to-date with latest literature, giving best of the technology and knowledge to Indian patients, ability to give final answer and overall raising the standard of Radiology in India has influenced me a lot. Their keen interest in teaching Radiology and the academic environment created by sir and madam has improved diagnostic abilities of many radiologists. This book is the reflection of their work. Without their guidance this would not have been possible.

I am very grateful to the academic environment at Jankharia Imaging with availability of books, journals, computers, good cases and above all able guidance so that I could complete this book. The high quality images used in this book are courtesy of Jankharia Imaging.

I was also grateful to 'Senior Sir' Dr. G.R. Jankharia and Dr. Bijal Jankharia for their encouragement and support. Thanks to my colleagues at JIC Drs–Pradeep Krishnan, Kishore Rajpal and Devang Desai for their help. Thanks to our brilliant technologist C.T. Kurian for his help with sequences and images.

I was made in KEM. I am grateful to Ravi Sir and the Radiology Department for instilling in me ability, confidence and values for patient care. I am also grateful to my PG teacher Dr. Malini Nadkarni for her constant encouragement.

My special thanks to Dr Manu Shroff, Sickkids, Toronto for his guidance and help.

I am lucky enough to have good senior friends like Titty Thomas (New York), Hemant Parmar (Michigan) and Vivek Sindhwani (Australia) who help and guide me. I am specially grateful to Hemant Parmar my 'guiding star'.

My sincere thanks to Shri Jitendar Pal Vij and Mr Tarun Duneja of Jaypee Brothers Medical Publishers (P) Ltd, New Delhi and Anshan, UK for publishing this work.

Last but not the least thanks to my wife Barkha and my family for their support and time.

Commonly Used Short Forms

ADC	Analog-to-Digital Converter/Apparrent Diffusion Coefficient
CEMRA	Contrast Enhanced MR Angiography
FOV	Field of View
FT	Fourier Transformation
GMR	Gradient Motion Rephasing/Nulling
GRE	Gradient Echo
IR	Inversion Recovery
LM	Longitudinal Magnetization
MTC	Magnetization Transfer Contrast
Nex	Number of Excitation (Averages of Acquisition)
NMV	Net Magnetization Vector
PD	Proton Density
RF	Radio-frequency
SAR	Specific Absorption Rate
SE	Spin Echo
SNR	Signal to Noise Ratio
TE	Time to Echo
TI	Time to Invert (Inversion Time)
TM	Middle Interval
TR	Time to Repeat
VENC	Velocity Encoding

Sequences Long Forms

BOLD	Blood Oxygen Level Dependant Imaging	**246**
CISS	Constructive Interference at Steady State	**74**
DESS	Double Echo in Steady State	**84**
EPI	Echo Plannar Imaging	**60**
FISP	Free Induction with Steady Precession	**65, 80**
FLAIR	Fluid Attenuated Inversion Recovery	**51, 70**
FLASH	Fast Low Angle Shot	**57, 68**
GMR	Gradient Moment Rephasing	**163**
GRASS	Gradient Recalled Acquisition in the Steady State	**65**
GRE	Gradient Echo Sequence	**54**
HASTE	Half Fourier Acquisition with Turbo Spin Echo	**81**
IPAT	Integrated Parallel Acquisition Technique	**62**
IR	Inversion Recovery Sequence	**49**
LOTA	Long-Term Averaging	**63**
MEDIC	Multi Echo Data Image Combination	**85**
MPRAGE	Magnetization Prepared Rapid Acquisition Gradient Echo	**75**
MTC	Magnetization Transfer Contrast	**250**
PC	Phase Contrast	**166**
RARE	Rapid Acquisition with Relaxation Enhancement	**58, 237**
ROPE	Respiratory Ordered Phase Encoding	**90**
SE	Spin Echo Sequence	**44**

SSFP	Steady State Free Precession	**57**
STE	Stimulated Echo	**59**
STEAM	Stimulated Echo Acquisition Method	**59, 201**
STIR	Short TI (inversion time) Inversion Recovery	**51, 76**
TOF	Time of Flight	**162**
TONE	Tilt Optimized Non-saturated Excitation	**64**
TRUFI	True FISP	**80**
TSE	Turbo Spin Echo	**47**
VIBE	Volume Interpolated Body Examination	**85**

Contents

Section I

1. Basic Principles 3
2. T1, T2 Relaxation and Other Parameters . 13
3. Instrumentation 25
4. Sequences I: Basic Principles 41
5. Sequences II: Few Common Sequences .. 67
6. Artifacts 87
7. MR Safety 105
8. MR Contrast Media 115
9. Principles of Interpretation:
   Neuroimaging 127
10. Principles of Interpretation:
    Body Imaging 143

Section II

11. MR Angiography 159
12. MR Diffusion 171
13. MR Perfusion 183
14. MR Spectroscopy 197
15. Cardiac MRI 219
16. MRCP 235
17. Miscellaneous MR Techniques 245

    Index 257

Section I

CHAPTER 1
Basic Principles

MRI MADE EASY (FOR BEGINNERS)

Four basic steps are involved in getting an MR image-
1. Placing the patient in the magnet
2. Sending radiofrequency (RF) pulse by coil
3. Receiving signals from the patient again by coil
4. Signals are sent to computers for complex processing to get image.

Now let us understand these steps at molecular level. Present MR imaging is based on proton imaging. Proton is a positively charged particle in the nucleus of every atom. Since hydrogen ion (H^+) has only one particle i.e. proton, it is equivalent to a proton.

How does this proton help in MR imaging?
Protons are positively charged and have rotatory movement called spin. Any charge, which moves, generates current. Every current has a small magnetic field around it. So every spinning proton has a small magnetic field around it.

Without any influence of external magnetic field protons in the patient's body move randomly in any direction. When external magnetic field is applied, i.e. patient is placed in the magnet, these randomly moving protons align and spin in the direction of external magnetic field. Some of them align parallel and some anti-parallel to the external magnetic field. When protons align, not only they rotate around themselves (called *spin*) but also their axis of rotation moves such that it forms a 'cone'. This movement of axis of rotation of proton is called as *precession* (Fig. 1.1).

BASIC PRINCIPLES 5

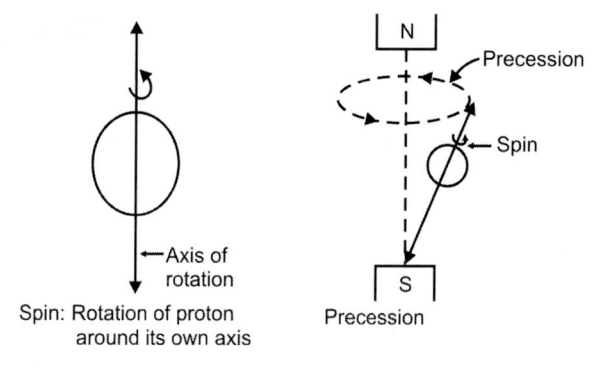

Fig. 1.1: Spin versus precession. Spin is rotation of protons around its own axis while precession is rotation of the axis itself under the influence of external magnetic field such that it forms a 'cone'

The number of precessions of proton per second is precession frequency in Hertz. Precession frequency is directly proportional to strength of external magnetic field. Stronger the external magnetic field, higher is precession frequency. This relationship is expressed by Larmor's equation–

$$W_o = yB_o$$

Where w_o = Precession frequency in Hz

B_o = Strength of external magnetic field in Tesla

Y = Gyromagnetic ratio, which is specific to particular nucleus

Precession frequency of hydrogen proton for 1 Tesla is 42 MHz and for 1.5 Tesla it is 64 MHz.

MAGNETIZATION

Now let us go one step further and understand what happens when protons align under influence of external

6 MRI MADE EASY (FOR BEGINNERS)

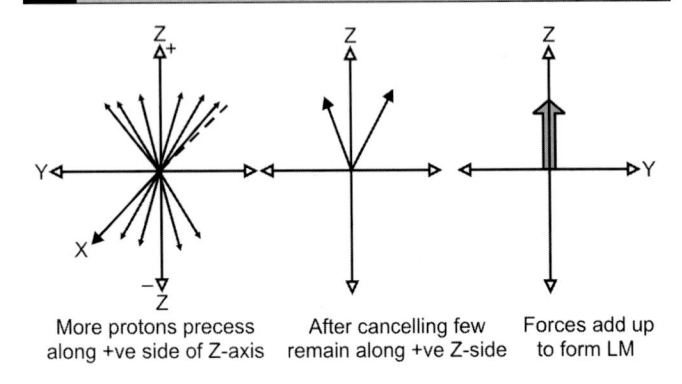

Fig. 1.2: Longitudinal magnetization

(Left) More protons precess along +ve side of Z-axis
(Middle) After cancelling few remain along +ve Z-side
(Right) Forces add up to form LM

magnetic field. For the orientation in space consider X, Y, and Z axes system. External magnetic field is directed along Z-axis. Conventionally, Z-axis is the long axis of the patient as well as bore of the magnet. Protons align parallel and anti-parallel to external magnetic field i.e. along positive and negative sides of Z-axis. Forces of protons on negative and positive side cancel each other. However, there are always more protons spinning on the positive side or parallel to Z-axis than negative side. So, after canceling each other few protons remain on positive side, which are not cancelled. Forces of these protons add up together to form a magnetic vector along Z-axis. This is **longitudinal magnetization** (Fig. 1.2).

Longitudinal magnetization along external magnetic field cannot be measured directly. For measurement it has to be transverse.

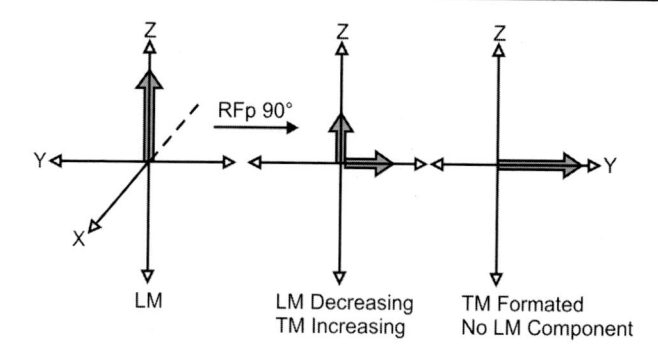

Fig. 1.3: Transverse magnetization. Magnetization vector is flipped in transverse plane by 90 degree RFp

Transverse Magnetization

As we discussed when patient is placed in the magnet, longitudinal magnetization vector forms along Z-axis and in the long axis of the patient. At this stage radiofrequency pulse is sent. Precessing protons pick up some energy from radiofrequency pulse. Some of these protons go to higher energy level and start precessing anti-parallel. This results in reduction in the magnitude of longitudinal magnetization. Forces of protons now add up to form a new magnetic vector in transverse (X-Y) plane. This is called as transverse magnetization (Fig. 1.3). In short, RF pulse causes longitudinal magnetization to reduce and establishes a new transverse magnetization.

For exchange of energy to occur between protons and RF pulse, precession frequency of protons should be same as RF pulse frequency. When RF pulse and protons have same frequency protons can pick up some energy from

8 MRI MADE EASY (FOR BEGINNERS)

RF pulse. This phenomenon is called as "resonance"—the R of MRI.

RF pulse not only causes protons to go to higher level but also makes them precess in step or in phase.

MR Signal

Transverse magnetization vector formed has a precession frequency. When it moves it produces electric current. The coils receive this current as MR signal (Fig. 1.4). Strength of the signal depends upon magnitude of the transverse magnetization. MR signals are Fourior Transformed into MR image by computers.

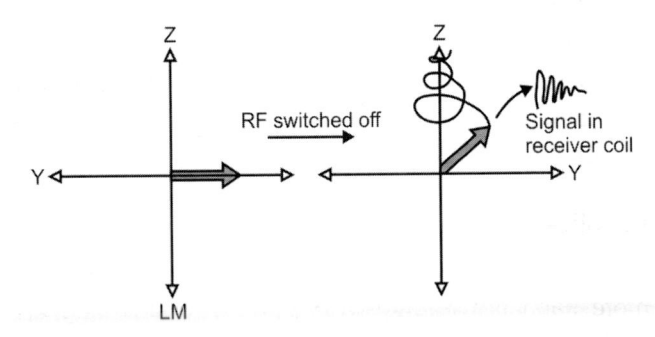

Fig. 1.4: MR signal. When RFp is switched off TM vector goes on reducing in its magnitude and LM goes on increasing. The resultant NMV formed by addition of these two (LM and TM vectors) gradually moves from transverse X-Y plane into vertical Z-axis. During this movement it produces current in receiver coil. This current received by the coil is MR signal

Revision

Once again revising those four steps of acquisition of MR image–

1. Patient is placed in the magnet
   All randomly moving protons in patent's body align and precess along external magnetic field. Longitudinal magnetization is formed long Z-axis.
2. RF pulse is sent
   Precessing protons pick up energy from RF pulse to go to higher energy level and precess in phase. This results in reduction in longitudinal magnetization and formation of transverse megnetization in X-Y plane.
3. MR signal
   Transverse magnetization vector precess and generates current. When RF pulse is switched off, this current produces signal in the coil.
4. Image formation
   Signal is transformed into image by complex mathematical process—Fourior Transformation by computers.

Localization of Signal

To localize from where in the body signals are coming three more magnetic fields are superimposed on main magnetic field along X, Y, and Z axes. These magnetic fields have different strength in varying location hence these fields are called "gradient fields" or simply "gradients".

The three gradients are:
1. Slice selection gradient
2. Phase encoding gradient
3. Frequency encoding gradient

10 MRI MADE EASY (FOR BEGINNERS)

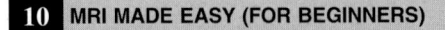

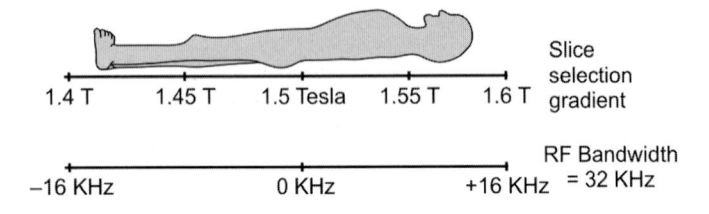

Fig. 1.5: Slice selection gradient

Slice Selection

Slice selection gradient has gradually increasing magnetic field strength from one end to another (Fig. 1.5). It determines slice position. Slice thickness is determined by bandwidth of RF pulse. Bandwidth is range of frequencies. Wider the bandwidth thicker is the slice.

To determine the point in a slice from where certain signal is coming, two more gradients—phase encoding and frequency encoding, are applied perpendicular to each other and perpendicular to slice selection gradient (Fig. 1.6).

Typically, for transverse or axial sections following are axes and gradients applied, even though X and Y axes can be varied.
1. Z-axis—Slice selection gradient
2. Y-axis—Frequency encoding gradient
3. X-axis—Phase encoding gradient.

In a usual sequence, slice selection gradient is sent at the time of RF pulse. Phase encoding gradient is turned on for a short-time after slice selection gradient. Frequency encoding or readout gradient is sent in the end at the time of signal reception.

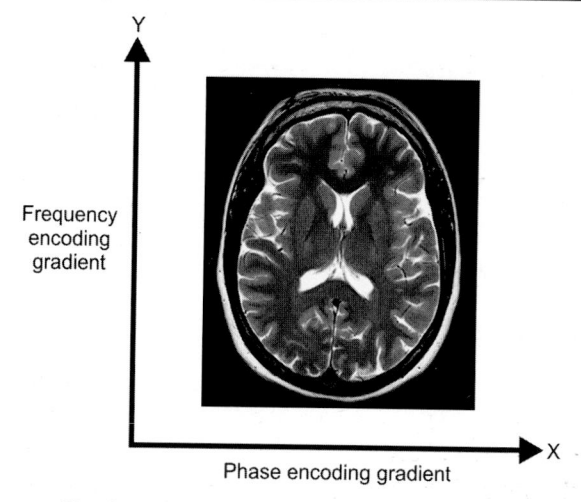

Fig. 1.6: Frequency and phase encoding gradients

Information from all three axes is sent to computers to get the particular point in that slice from which the signal is coming.

Why Proton Only?

Other nuclei can be used for MR imaging. Requirement is that they should have spin and should have odd number of protons in the nucleus. Hence, theoretically 13C, 19F, 23Na, 31P can be used for MR imaging.

Hydrogen atom has only one proton. Hence H^+ ion is equivalent to a proton. Hydrogen ions are present in abundance in body water. H^+ gives best and most intense signal among all nuclei.

CHAPTER 2

T1, T2 Relaxation and Other Parameters

14 MRI MADE EASY (FOR BEGINNERS)

Relaxation means recovery of protons back towards equilibrium after been disturbed by RF excitation. Relaxation times of protons and heterogeneous distribution of tissue-proton densities determine the contrast in an MR image.

We have seen that RF pulse causes LM to reduce and TM to form. What happens when RF pulse is switched off?

When RF pulse is switched off TM reduces, which is called as Transverse Relaxation and LM increases, which is called as Longitudinal Relaxation.

The net magnetization vector (NMV) is the sum of two vectors in different planes (like LM and TM vector) represented as single vector in a plane midway between the two.

LONGITUDINAL RELAXATION (FIG. 2.1)

When RF pulse is switched off, protons start losing their energy. This energy is given to surrounding or lattice, hence this is also called as 'spin-lattice' relaxation. As protons

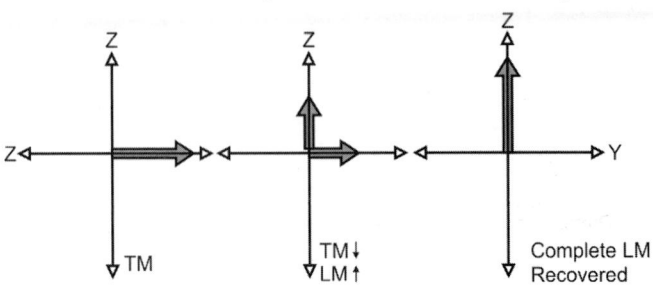

Fig. 2.1: Longitudinal relaxation

T1, T2 RELAXATION AND OTHER PARAMETERS

lose their energy, the magnitude of LM increases. When curve is plotted of LM magnitude against time, it is called as T1 curve.

T1 is the time taken for LM to recover after RF pulse is switched off, to original value.

TRANSVERSE RELAXATION (FIG. 2.2)

Protons which were precessing in phase because of RF pulse, start losing phase after RF pulse is switched off. This going out of phase of protons results into gradual decrease in the magnitude of TM and is termed as Transverse relaxation. The time taken by TM to reduce to its original value is transversal relaxation time or T2. Longitudinal and transversal relaxations are different and independent processes because underlying mechanisms are different.

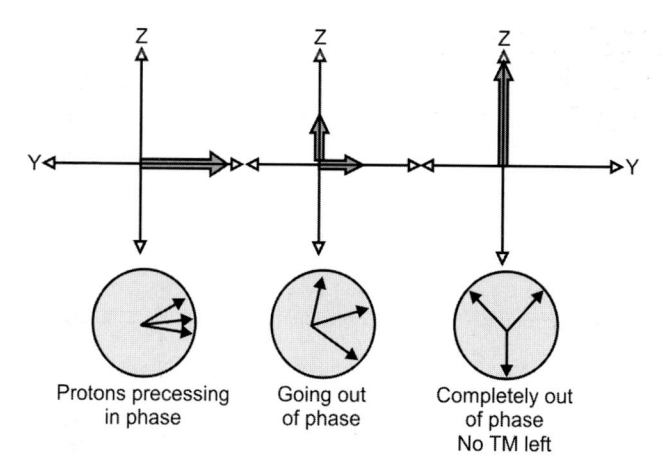

Fig. 2.2: Transverse relaxation

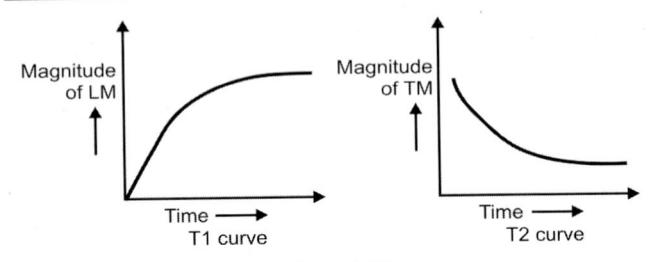

Fig. 2.3: T1 and T2 curves

T1

T1 is the time taken by LM to recover after RF pulse is switched off, to original value. This is not exact time, but it is a 'constant'. T1 is the time when LM reaches back to 63% of its original value. 1/T1 is longitudinal relaxation rate (Fig. 2.3).

T1 depends upon tissue composition, structure and surroundings. If lattice (surrounding matter) has magnetic field, which fluctuates at Larmor frequency, transfer of thermal energy from protons to the lattice is easy and fast. Protons in such surrounding have shorter T1. However, in water since water molecules move too rapidly. This increases time taken to transfer energy from protons to lattice. Hence water has long T1.

Fatty acids have frequency near Larmor frequency so there is fast energy transfer from protons to lattice. Hence fat has short T1.

T1 is longer in stronger magnetic field.

T2

T2 is time taken by TM to disappear. Again like T1 it is a constant and not exact time. It is the time taken by TM

T1, T2 RELAXATION AND OTHER PARAMETERS

to reduce to 37% of its original value. 1/T2 is transverse relaxation rate.

T2 depends on inhomogeneity of external magnetic field and inhomogeneity of local magnetic field within tissues. As water molecules move very fast, their magnetic fields fluctuate fast. These fluctuating magnetic fields cancel each other. So there are no big differences in magnetic field strength inside a tissue. Because of lack of much inhomogeneity protons stay in step for a long time resulting into long T2 for water.

If liquid is impure and has larger molecules, they move at slower rate. This maintains inhomogeneity of magnetic field. As a result protons go out of phase very fast. Hence impure liquids, larger molecules have short T2, e.g. Fat has shorter T2.

TR and TE

A typical spin-echo sequence consists of 90 degree pulse followed by 180 degree pulse, at the end of which echo (signal) is received (Fig. 2.4).

TR (Time to Repeat) is the time interval between start of one RF pulse and start of next RF pulse. Typically in spin-echo sequence time interval between beginnings of 90 degree pulses is TR.

TE (Time to Echo) is the time interval between start of RF pulse and reception of the echo (signal).

Short TR and short TE gives T1-weighted images.
Long TR and long TE gives T2-weighted images.
Long TR and short TE gives proton density images.

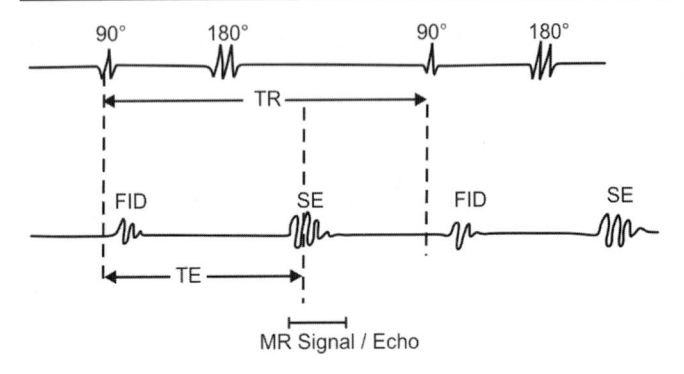

Fig. 2.4: Spin-echo (SE) sequence

Typically long TR is >1500 ms (millisecond) and short TR is <500 ms. However, there is no fixed range. Short TE is around 15-20 ms and long is above 70-75 ms.

TR is always higher than TE.

TI

TI is Time of Inversion. It is the time between inverting 180 degree pulse and 90 degree pulse in Inversion recovery (IR) sequence. TI determines contrast IR sequence.

T1-WEIGHTED IMAGE

LM is one of the determinants of strength of MR signal. Stronger the LM more will be the magnitude of TM after 90 degree pulse that results into stronger signal. If T1 is short, there is early or maximum regain of LM after RF pulse is switched off. So, if next RF pulse is sent, TM will be stronger and resultant signal will also be stronger. So,

T1, T2 RELAXATION AND OTHER PARAMETERS 19

material with short T1 have bright signal on T1 weighted images.

How do we make images T1-weighted?
This is done by keeping TR short. If TR is long the tissues with long T1 will also regain maximum LM giving stronger TM with next RF pulse and stronger signal. This will result in no difference between tissues with different T1. So in T1-W images differences in signal intensity in tissues is due to their difference in T1 (Figs 2.5A and B).

T2-WEIGHTED IMAGE

Tissues with long T2 are bright on T2-W images. Longer the T2 of any tissue, larger TM will remain for more time. This will lead to stronger signal, because stronger TM gives stronger signal.

How do we make images T2-weighted?
With short TE, difference between tissue A and B (Figs 2.6A and B) will be less pronounced. With long TE signal difference between A and B, i.e. tissues with long (A) and short (B) T2 will be more. So, image with long TE is T2-weighted since signal difference between tissues (contrast) is determined by T2 of tissues.

However, shorter the TE, stronger is signal. So it has to be trade off between signal intensity and T2 weighting.

PROTON DENSITY (PD) IMAGE

Contrast in the image is determined by density of protons in the tissue. T1 effect is reduced by keeping long TR and T2 effect is reduced by keeping TE short. Hence long TR and short TE gives PD-weighted image (Fig. 2.7).

20   **MRI MADE EASY (FOR BEGINNERS)**

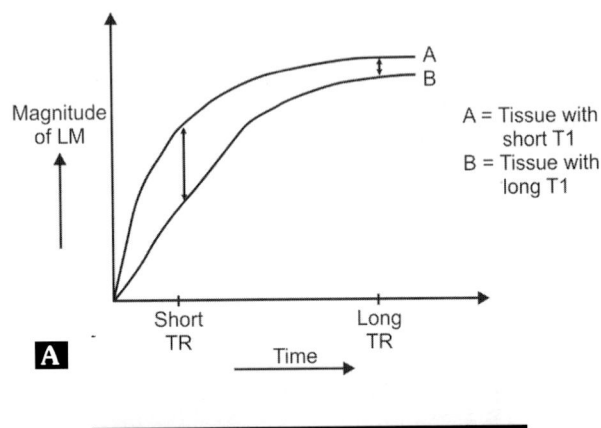

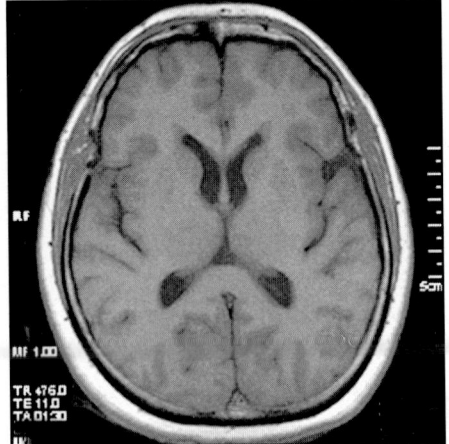

Figs 2.5A and B: T1-weighted image

A. At short TR the difference between LM of tissue A (with short T1) and of tissue B (long T1) is more so the difference in signal intensity of A and B (contrast) is more. At long TR difference between signals from A and B is less. So at short TR image contrast is obtained because of T1 differences of tissues. Hence it is T1-weighted image
B. T1-weighted axial image of brain: CSF is dark, white matter is brighter than gray matter and scalp fat is bright because of short T1

T1, T2 RELAXATION AND OTHER PARAMETERS

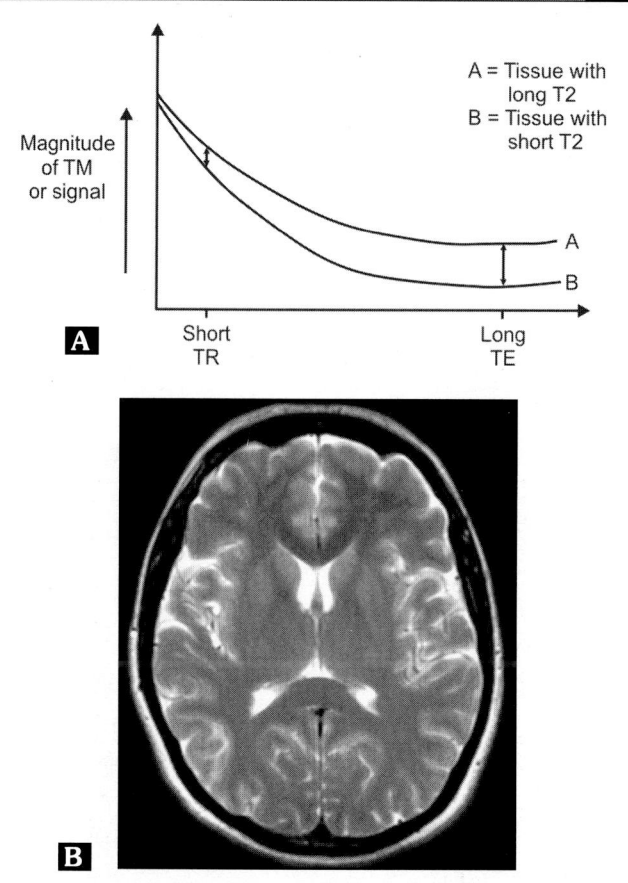

Fig. 2.6: T2-weighted image

A. Tissue B has short T2, which results into early loss of magnitude of TM and reduction in signal. At short TE there is not much difference between TM of A and B. At long TE signal difference between A and B is more because tissue B will have less signal intensity than tissue A. Since the image contrast is because of differences in T2 of tissues, it is T2-weighted image.
B. T2-weighted axial image of brain: CSF is bright, white matter is darker than gray matter.

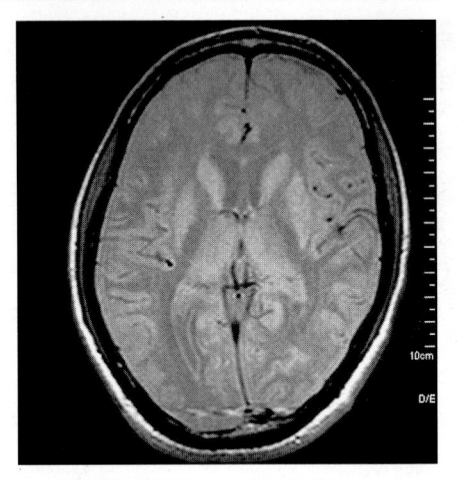

Fig. 2.7: Proton-density image

OTHER PARAMETERS OF SCANNING

1. Matrix: Matrix consists of rows and columns of pixels. Matrix of 256 x 256 means the image has 256 rows and 256 columns of pixels. More the size of matrix better is the resolution. However, it increases scanning time. For the same FOV if matrix is increased pixel size will reduce. Smaller the pixels better is resolution (Fig. 2.8).
2. SNR: Signal to noise ratio improves with number of averages, FOV, surface and phased array coils.
3. Number of excitations (average): More the number of acquisitions better will be SNR but it increases scan time.
4. Flip angle: It is the angle by which longitudinal magnetisation vector is rotated away from Z-axis by

T1, T2 RELAXATION AND OTHER PARAMETERS 23

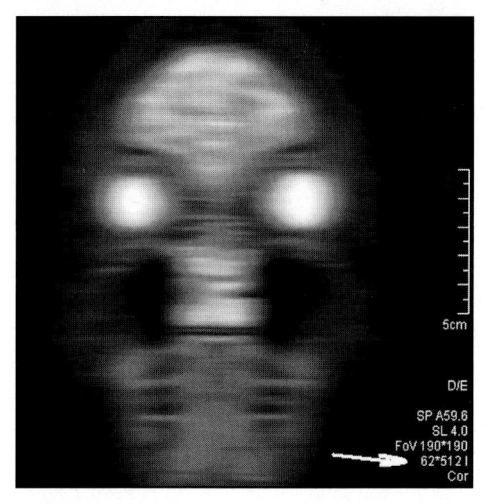

Fig. 2.8: Effect of matrix on image. By mistake the technician performing the scan forgot to type 0 and the matrix became 62 × 512 instead of 620 × 512! See the effect on the image, it is blurred

RF pulse. Shorter the flip angle less will be scanning time. Shorter flip angles are used in Gradient Echo sequences.

5. FOV: It is the area from which signals are acquired. It is selected as per requirement of the part under examination by technologist. Increasing FOV improves SNR, reduces resolution.
6. Bandwidth: Bandwidth is the range of frequencies. Reducing receive bandwidth increases SNR. However, it also increases chemical shift and minimum TE that can be used.

IMAGING TIME:
$$aT = TR \times N^* \times Nex$$

Where aT = Acquisition time
 TR = Time to repeat
 N* = Number of pixels (matrix)
 Nex = Number of excitation (to improve signal to noise ratio multiple excitations are averaged)

How to reduce imaging time?
1. As you can see from equation, decreasing TR will reduce acquisition time. But there are problems with reduced TR: 1. Images become more T1-weighted, 2. 180 degree pulse in spin echo sequence cannot be used.
2. Reducing number of pixels and number of excitation will reduce the time but it also reduces SNR and resolution.
3. Using smaller flip angle—10-35 degrees instead of 90 degree RF pulse as used in gradient echo imaging.
4. Multislice imaging: While waiting for TR of one slice to go by calculations, measurements of other slices done.
5. Use of gadolinium: Gadolinium reduces T1 leading to reduced TR and reduced time.

CHAPTER 3
Instrumentation

INTRODUCTION

In this chapter we will discuss about equipment required to get MR image. Basic four components make MR system.
1. The magnet to produce external magnetic field
2. Gradients to localise the signal
3. Transmitter and receiver coils for RF pulses
4. Computer system.

MAGNETISM

Magnetism is fundamental property of matter. All substances possess some form of magnetism. Degree of magnetism depends upon the magnetic susceptibility of the atom, which make the substance.

Magnetic susceptibility is the ability of the substance to get affected by external magnetic field and is related to electron configuration of the atom. Depending on the magnetic susceptibility, i.e. substance's response to magnetic field, substances can be paramagnetic, diamagnetic or ferromagnetic.

Paramagnetism

Paramagnetic substances have unpaired electrons within the atom. This results into a small magnetic field around them called magnetic moment. When external magnetic field applied, these moment add together and align in the direction of external magnetic field. Thus paramagnetic substances affect external magnetic field in positive way by attraction towards the field resulting in a local increase in magnetic field. Examples of paramagnetic substances are gadolinium, oxygen, melanin.

Diamagnetism

Diamagnetic substances react in opposite way when external magnetic field is applied. They are repelled by the magnetic field. Thus diamagnetic substances have negative magnetic susceptibility and show slight decrease in magnetic field strength within the sample.

Ferromagnetism

Ferromagnetic substances, when come in contact with a magnetic field, they get strongly attracted. Moreover, they retain their magnetism even when external magnetic field is removed. Such substances are used to make permanent magnet. The magnetic field in permanent magnet can be hundred or even thousands of times greater than applied external magnetic field. Examples of ferromagnetic substances are Iron, Cobalt and Nickel.

MAGNETIC FIELD STRENGTH

Magnetic field strength is expressed by notation 'B', the primary field as B0 and the secondary field as B1. The units of magnetic field strength are Gauss and Tesla. Tesla was Father of Alternating Current and Gauss was German mathematician.

$$1 \text{Tesla} = 10 \text{ kG} = 10,000 \text{ Gauss}$$

Gauss is a measure of low magnetic field strength. Earth's magnetic field strength is approximately 0.6 G.

MR systems used for clinical purpose have strength ranging from 0.2 to 3 Tesla. Field strengths higher than 3T are used for research purposes. As strength increases resolution increases. Advanced MR applications like Spectroscopy, functional MRI, cardiac MR are possible only on higher field strengths like 1.5 T.

MAGNETS

Three types of magnets are in use for clinical MRI machines.
1. Permanent magnet
2. Electromagnet
3. Superconducting magnet

Permanent Magnet

Permanent magnet is made up of ferromagnetic substances. Usually MR magnets are made up of *alnico*, which is alloy of aluminium, nickel and cobalt.

Permanent magnets do not require power supply and are of low cost. The magnetic field of permanent magnet is directed vertically (Fig. 3.1). Open MRI is possible with permanent magnet, which are useful in claustrophobic patients. Magnetic field strength achievable with permanent magnet is low in the range of 0.2 to 0.5 Tesla. Hence they have low SNR, low resolution and higher applications like spectroscopy cannot be done on them.

Electromagnets

These are based on principle of electromagnetism. The law of electromagnetism states that moving electric charge

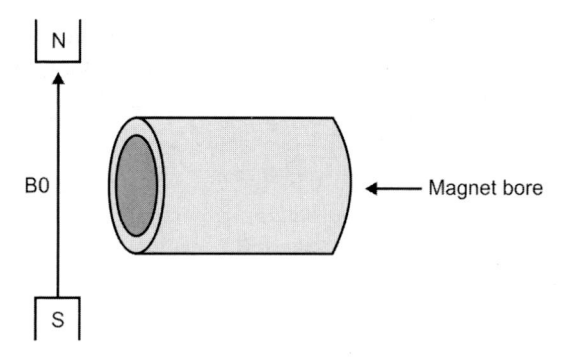

Fig. 3.1: Magnetic field: The magnetic field of the permanent magnet is vertically directed perpendicular to the long axis of the bore

induces magnetic field around it. If a current is passed through a wire, a magnetic field is created around that wire. The strength of the resultant magnetic field is proportional to the amount of current moving through the wire.

When a wire is looped like a spring (coil) and current is passed through it, the magnetic field generated is directed along the long axis of the coil. Magnets made of such coils are called solenoid or resistive electromagnets.

All wires at normal temperature tend to resist the passage of current. As the resistance increases, current decreases with resultant reduction in field strength. To get a homogenous field current must be steady and stable. The heat generated during this process is removed by running cooled water through tubes passing over the ends of the coil. Because of power required and cooling requirements, the field strength obtained with electromagnets is limited to 0.2 to 0.3 Tesla. This limits SNR and spectroscopy application. Even though capital cost is low operational cost is high for electromagnets because enormous power is required. However, electromagnets are easy to install and can readily be turned on and off inexpensively.

Superconducting Magnets

Some metals like mercury or Niobium-Titanium alloy lose their electric resistance at very low temperature and become superconductors. As discussed in electromagnets as resistance decreases current increases. And as current increases magnetic field strength increases. Therefore in superconducting magnet higher field strength is achieved by completely eliminating resistance. Moreover, once superconductor wires or coils are energised the current continues in a loop as long as the superconducting wire is maintained below the critical temperature. There is no power loss and continuous power supply is not required to maintain magnetic field.

Structure of Superconducting Magnet (Fig. 3.2)

Superconducting wires
These are made up of Nb/Ti alloy. This alloy becomes superconducting at 10K (kelvin) and produces magnetic field when current is passed through it. A wire containing filaments of Nb/Ti alloy embedded in a copper matrix is wound tightly and precisely on an insulated aluminium

INSTRUMENTATION

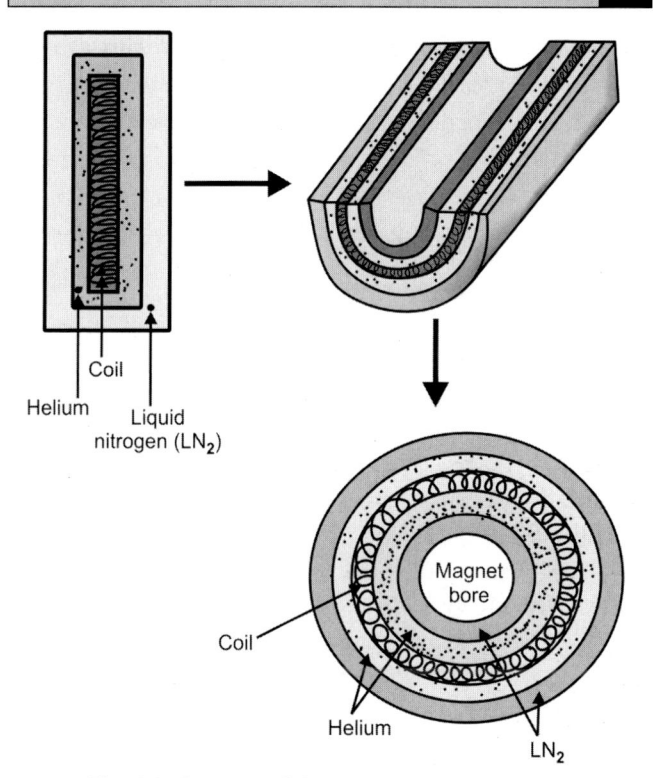

Fig. 3.2: Structure of the superconducting magnet

bore tube and fixed in place with a viscous, high thermal conductivity epoxy binder. There are thousands of turns of the wire, which may be 30 Kilometer long. Since it is not possible to wound, the coil with a single continuos strand, coil has several interconnecting joints.

Helium

The coil of superconducting material is cooled to 4K (-269 degree celcium) by liquid helium, which surrounds coil all around. Because of smaller heat leaks into the system, *cryogens* like helium steadily boil off. This boil off is reduced by much cheap liquid nitrogen. However, helium should be replenished on regular basis, usually every six months.

Liquid Nitrogen and Radiation Shield

The can of liquid helium is surrounded by cooled liquid nitrogen and radiation shields. This prevents any heat exchange between helium and the surrounding. Nitrogen boils at 80 degree K and much cheaper than helium. The liquid nitrogen and radiation shields reduce evapouration of liquid helium to 0.3 liter per hour.

Starting the Magnet

When magnet is started first time, it is done in a particular way or sequence. First, superconducting coil is cooled to -269 degree Celsius by helium and liquid nitrogen. Then the magnet is energised by delivering current from external power source to superconducting wire (coil). This process is called *ramping*. Once desirable level of current is achieved, power supply is cut off. The current continues to circulate through the coil. The current and the magnetic field produced by it remains constant subjected only to minor changes.

Quench

Quench is discharge or loss of magnetic field of superconducting magnet. This occurs because of increased resistance in the superconducting coil, which results in heat formation. This heat in turn causes cryogens to evaporate.

This sets in a vicious cycle, which ultimately results in increased temperature, increased resistance, evaporation of all cryogens and complete loss of magnetic field. Triggering factor to increase in resistance could be minor motion of wire in the coil or flux jumping, which results in heat production.

Rarely, quench can be deliberately performed to save patient's life. This is done for example in situation where oxygen cylinder accidentally traps the patient inside the magnet.

All MR systems should have vent to pass helium to outside environment in case quench occurs. Helium released inside the scan room can replace the oxygen completely and can cause asphyxia. It also produces increased pressure in the scan room, which may prevent opening of the door. Every scan room should have oxygen monitor that will alarm if oxygen level falls below critical level.

To start the magnet after quench, cryogens are filled and wires are cooled. Then ramping is done till desirable level of magnetic field is achieved.

Magnetic Field Homogeneity

Magnetic field should be uniform all over its extent to get correct information (signal) from the patient. Even though magnetic field is more or less uniform there might be minor inhomogeneity. The process of making the magnetic field homogenous is called as "*shimming*". This process is necessary because of the difficulty of winding a perfect coil, slight current densities within the wire and presence of metal within the environment, which leads to magnetic field inhomogeneity.

Shimming can be active or passive. Passive shimming is done by keeping metal pieces, called shim plates, in the field to oppose the inhomogeneity.

Active shimming is done by passing current through the gradient coils, which generates small magnetic field gradients superimposed on main magnetic field (B0). These coils are called shim coils. Shim coils make field homogenous by adding or substracting from the field at desired points. Shim coils can be resistive windings located within the room temperature bore of the magnet or superconducting windings located within the helium vessel.

Homogeneity is expressed as parts per million (ppm). Homogeneity of 10 ppm is sufficient for routine spin echo imaging. However, for proton spectroscopy a highly homogenous field of 0.1 ppm is required to be able to detect metabolites with smaller chemical shift differences.

Shielding

The stray magnetic field outside the bore of the magnet is known as *fringe field*. This stray field can cross-conventional walls, floors or ceilings and can potentially harmful to patients with pacemakers, for monitoring devices, and other magnetically-activated devices present nearby. To prevent this MR system is shielded by two processes:
1. Passive shielding, and
2. Active shielding.

Passive shielding is done by lining the wall of MR room by steel or copper. This chamber so shielded is called as *'Faraday cage'*.

Active shielding uses additional solenoid magnet outside the cryogen bath that restricts the Bo lines to a acceptable location. However, active shielding is an expensive alternative.

GRADIENTS

Gradients or gradient coils are used to vary magnetic field strength over the extent of magnetic field. Gradient system consists of three sets of coils that produce field with changing strength in X, Y, Z directions. Three gradients are used for slice selection, phase encoding and frequency encoding when applied in three directions perpendicular to each other.

How gradient coils are produced?
Magnetic field strength is proportional to the amount of current passed through the loop of wire, number of loops in wire, the size of the loop and how closely the loops are spaced. By changing these parameters coil can be produced, which increases or decreases magnetic field strength in particular direction.

Gradient strength (stiffness) is measured in units of G/cm or mT/m. This means that the magnetic field strength changes by one Gauss over each centimeter or 10 milliTesla over each meter. Stronger gradients (15 or 20 mT/m) allow high speed and high resolution imaging.

Gradient strength has effect on slice thickness and FOV that can be used. For a constant bandwidth, weaker gradient will produce thicker slice and stronger gradient will produce thinner slice.

Quality of gradient system depends on gradient linearity and their rise and fall time. In typical spin-echo imaging slice selection gradient is on for 3 ms, the phase encoding gradient for 4 ms and frequency encoding (readout) gradient for 8 ms.

Problem with gradient system is generation of eddy current. Eddy current degrade the homogeneity of the magnetic field. They also cause heat production, which results in evapouration of cryogens. Various methods are used to minimise eddy current.

Gradient coils are located coaxially in the room temperature compartment of the magnet bore.

Apart from localization gradients are used for gradient echo sequence. Gradients are used for spoiling or rewinding transverse magnetization. Gradients are used to rephase the protons when they are going out of phase after RF pulse is switched off. Thus eliminating 180 degree pulse and making the gradient echo sequence much faster.

RADIOFREQUENCY COILS

A loop of wire is coil. Radiofrequency (RF) coils are used to transmit RF pulse into the patient and to receive the signals from the patient. RF coils can be transmitters, receivers or both transmitter and receiver then it is called as *transceiver*. Energy is transmitted in the form of short

INSTRUMENTATION

intense bursts of radiofrequencies known as radiofrequency pulses. This RF pulses cause phase coherence and flip some of the protons from a low energy states to high energy states. RF pulse that causes net magnetization vector to flip by 90 degree is called as 90 degree RF pulse. Rotating TM vector induces current in the receiver coil, which forms *signal*.

Various types of RF coils are:
1. Body coil
2. Head coil
3. Surface or local coil
4. Phased array coil
5. Solenoid coil
6. Helmholtz coil

Head and body coils are volume coils and are transceivers. They cover larger area and give uniform SNR over the entire imaging volume. However, SNR is lower than other types of coils. They also act as transmitters for surface or local coils.

Surface coils improve SNR significantly when used to image structures near the surface of the patient. Area covered is sensitive volume covered by the coil. Signal drops as the distance of the structure increased from the coil. Body coil acts as transmitter for surface coil, which are receiver only. Various surface or local coils are designed as per requirement for the particular parts. Examples are flex coils that can be wrapped around knee, shoulder and ankle. There are orbit and carotid coils. Local coils can

38 MRI MADE EASY (FOR BEGINNERS)

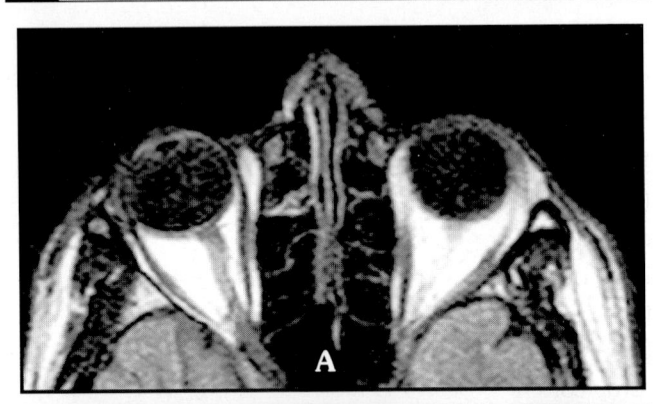

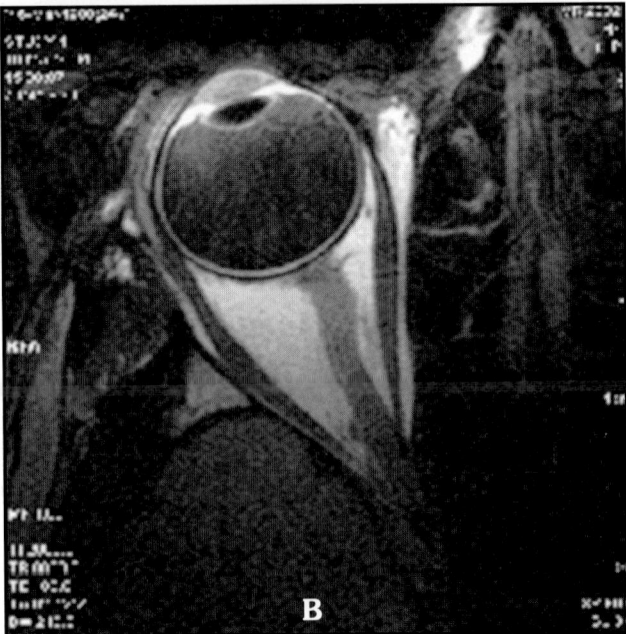

Figs 3.3A and B: Surface versus volume coil. Note the increased resolution and details in image with orbit coil (B) as compared to the image with head coil (A). Also note decreased signal beyond the orbital apex

be endoluminal for example rectal coil for prostate imaging. All these coils give images with high SNR and high resolution.

Phased Array coils combine advantages of surface coils (increased SNR and resolution) and volume coils (increased coverage). They consist of multiple small coils. The signal input of each coil is separately received and processed and then combined to form single larger FOV. There could be four (4 channel) or six (6 channel) small coils in phased array coils. Phased array coils are used in body imaging, spine, pelvis, cardiac, MRCP and other imaging (Figs 3.3A and B).

COMPUTERS AND ACCESSORIES

This is the last component of MR system. Computer system control every application. They perform functions of data collection and manipulation, image viewing, storage, retrieval and documentation.

CHAPTER 4

Sequences I: Basic Principles

INTRODUCTION

A pulse sequence is interplay of various parameters leading to a complex cascade of events with RF pulses and gradients to from a MR image (Fig. 4.1).

So pulse sequence is a time chart of interplay of:
1. Patient's net longitudinal magnetisation
2. Transmission of RF pulses (90, 180 degree or any degree)
3. X, Y and Z gradient activation for localisation and acquisition of signal (echo)
4. K-space filling with acquired signals or echoes.

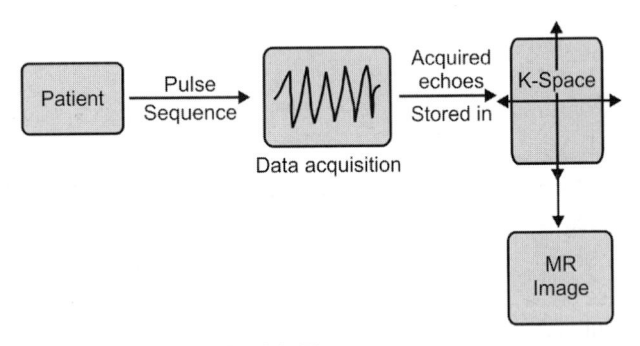

Fig. 4.1: The sequence

k-SPACE

k-space is an imaginary space which represents raw data matrix. After acquisition all signals are stored in k-space. This raw data from k-space is then used to reconstruct image by Fourier Transformation.

k-space has two axes. Horizontal axis represents the phase axis and is centered in the middle of several

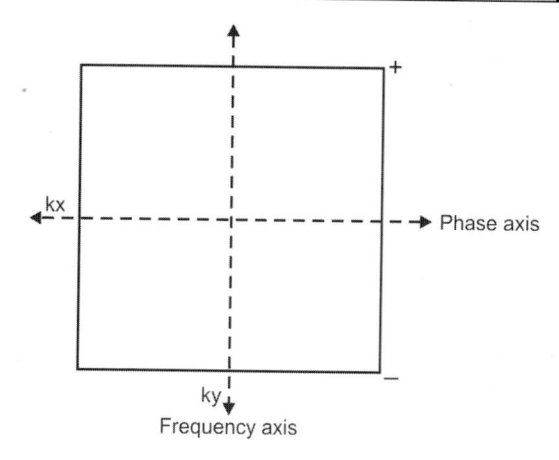

Fig. 4.2: k-space

horizontal lines. The frequency axis of k-space is vertical and is perpendicular to phase axis (Fig. 4.2).

Signal is filled in k-space as horizontal line. The number of lines of k-space that are filled, is determined by the number of different phase encoding steps. If 128 different phase encoding steps are selected then 128 lines of k-space are filled to complete the scan.

In conventional spin-echo imaging one line of k-space is filled every TR. If matrix size is 128 × 128 then 128 TRs will be required to form an image. K-space is filled from center to periphery. Two halves of k-space- right and left or upper and lower are exact symmetric conjugate and represent same information. This fact is used to manipulate k-space sampling (partial sampling) to get same image in less time. In fast imaging like HASTE only half of k-space is filled. In ultrafast Echo Planar Imaging (EPI) all the k-space lines required to form an image are filled in a single TR, thus reducing the scanning time in seconds.

Center part of k-space represents contrast of the image. Periphery corresponds with resolution and fine details.

The parameters will be discussed during particular sequences. Let's first start with the basic classification of sequences.

Pulse sequences can broadly be divided into following categories:
1. Spin-echo sequence (SE)
a. Conventional SE
b. Fast/turbo SE
2. Inversion recovery (IR)
3. Gradient echo sequence (GRE)
4. Ultrafast sequences like EPI.

SPIN-ECHO PULSE SEQUENCE (SE)

It consists of 90 and 180 degree pulses. Excitatory 90 degree pulse flips net magnetisation vector by 90 degree from along Z-axis into transverse X-Y plane. When 90 degree pulse is switched off, protons start dephasing and amount of TM magnetisation reduces. At this stage second pulse of 180 degree is sent. This 180 degree pulse also called as rephasing pulse, brings protons back into phase. This rephasing results into increased magnitude of TM and echo or signal is received by the receiver coil. This is called as spin-echo. This is basic design of SE sequence. The

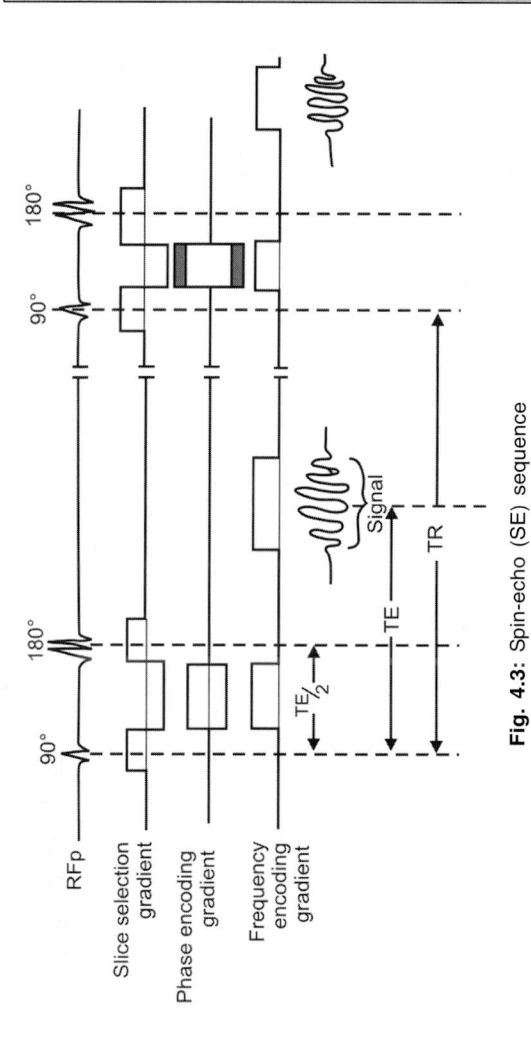

SEQUENCES I: BASIC PRINCIPLES 45

Fig. 4.3: Spin-echo (SE) sequence

time between two 90 degree pulses is called as TR (Time to Repeat). The time between 90 degree pulse and reception of echo (signal) is TE (Time to Echo) (Fig. 4.3).

As far as localisation gradients are concerned, slice selection gradient is turned on when RF is sent. Phase encoding gradient is turned on between excitation (90 degree) pulse and signal measurement. Phase encoding gradient has different strength for each TR. Frequency encoding also called as read out gradient is turned on during signal measurement.

In conventional SE sequence one line of k-space is filled per TR.

SE is mother of all sequences and forms basis for understanding all other sequences. It is used in almost all examinations. T1-weighted images are useful for demonstrating anatomy. Since tissues that are diseased, are generally more edematous and or vascular, they appear bright on T2-weighted images. Therefore, T2-weighted images demonstrates pathology well.

Modification of SE

SE sequence can be modified to have more than one echo per TR. This is done by sending more than one 180 pulses after the excitatory 90 degree pulse. Each 180 degree pulse obtains one echo. The PD + T2 double echo sequence (Fig. 4.4) is an example of such modified SE sequence. In this sequence TR is long. After first 180 degree pulse since TE is short, image will be proton density weighted (long TR, short TE). After second 180 pulse TE will be

Fig. 4.4: PD + T2 double echo sequence

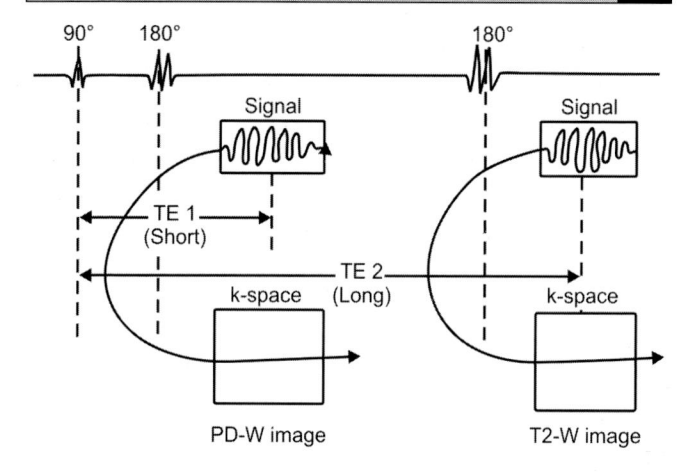

One line in separate k-spaces per TR

long, T2-W image (long TR, long TE) will be obtained. Both these echoes contribute separate k-space lines in two different k-spaces.

Turbo Spin-Echo Sequence

When multiple 180 degree rephasing pulses are sent after 90 degree pulse, it is called as multi spin-echo or Turbo spin-echo sequence (Fig. 4.5). In this sequence multiple echoes obtained per TR; one echo with each 180 degree pulse. All the echoes are used to fill single or common k-space. Since k-space is filled much faster with multiple echoes filled in single TR the scanning speed increases considerably.

Fig. 4.5: Turbo spin-echo sequence

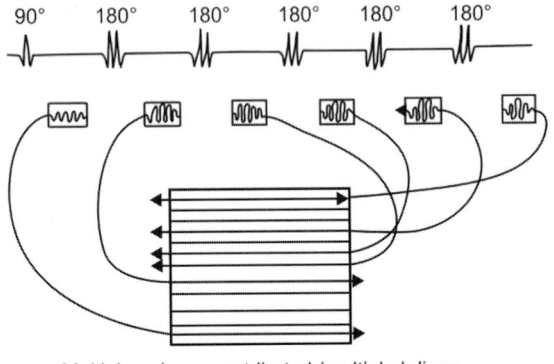

Multiple echoes contributed (multiple k-lines filled) to single k-space per TR

Turbo factor: Turbo factor is number of 180 degree pulses after each 90 degree pulse. It is also called as **echo train length**. The amplitude of signal (echo) generated from the multiple refocusing 180 degree pulses varies since TE goes on increasing. TE effective is that TE, which fills the center of k-space. It gives maximum amplitude.

Short turbo factor decreases effective TE, increases T1 weighting. However, it increases scan time. Long turbo factor increases effective TE, increases T2 weighting and reduces scan time. However, it reduces number of slices per TR and increases image blurring.

Usefulness of Multi-Spin-Echo Sequence

Image contrast of TSE is similar to SE sequence. Therefore, these sequences are useful in most clinical applications as SE sequence. Added advantage is greatly reduced scan time such that acquisition can be completed in single breath-hold. HASTE and RARE are examples of TSE, which will be discussed in MRCP.

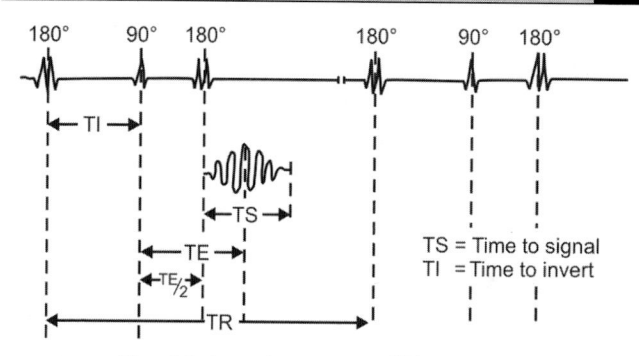

Fig. 4.6: Inversion recovery (IR) sequence

Inversion Recovery (IR) Sequence

IR sequence consists of an inverting 180 degree pulse followed by 90 degree excitation pulse followed by rephasing 180 degree pulse (Fig. 4.6).

Inverting 180 pulse flips LM from positive side of Z-axis to negative side of Z-axis to saturate NMV fully. After inverting 180 degree pulse is switched off NMV begins to relax or LM gradually builds back along positive side of Z-axis. After a time 90 degree excitatory pulse is applied. This time between inversion 180 degree and excitatory 90 degree pulse is called as TI- Time to invert. TI is the main determinant of contrast in IR sequences. The 90 degree pulse flips NMV into transverse plane. When it is switched off spins start dephasing and magnitude of TM reduces, 180 degree rephasing pulse is applied to get the signal, same way as in SE sequence. Rephasing can also be done by gradients instead of 180 degree pulse.

Why do we use inverting 180 degree pulse? What do we achieve?

The inversion 180 degree pulse flips NMV along negative side of Z-axis. This saturates fat and water completely at the beginning of each 90 degree pulse. When 90 degree excitatory pulse is applied after NMV has relaxed through the transverse plane, contrast in the image depends on the amount of longitudinal recovery, as in SE sequence. However, image in IR is more heavily T1-weighted because of 180 degree pulse achieving full saturation and large contrast difference between fat and water. Apart from getting heavily T1-weighted images to demonstrate anatomy, IR sequence also used to suppress particular tissue depending on TI. IR sequence also can be used in post-contrast imaging as they enhance signals from tissues taking up contrast.

Tissue Suppression

If TI corresponds with time the tissue takes to recover after 180 degree inversion pulse from full inversion to transverse plane, there will not be any longitudinal magnetisation. So, when 90 degree pulse is applied there is no TM, i.e. no signal. IR sequences are thus used to suppress certain tissues by changing TI. The TI required to null the signal from a tissue is 0.69 times T1 relaxation time of that tissue.

SEQUENCES I: BASIC PRINCIPLES

Types of IR Sequences

IR sequences can be of short, medium and long TI.

Short TI is 80 to 150 ms and example is STIR. Medium TI ranges from 200 to 800 ms and examples are MPRAGE and turbo FLASH. Long TI ranges from 1500 to 2500 ms and example is FLAIR.

Short TI IR Sequence STIR (Figs 4.7A and B)

When 90 degree pulse is applied at short TI, LM for all or virtually all tissues is negative. This results in increased sensitivity to T1 and T2 changes. Because many pathologies increase both T1 and T2, addition of these two types of contrast in STIR gives high net tissue contrast. By choosing particular TI, tissue can be suppressed. In short TI IR sequences fat is suppressed since fat has short T1. Most of the pathologies appear bright on STIR making them easier to pick up.

Long TI IR Sequence FLAIR (Figs 4.8A and B)

When 90 degree pulse is applied at long TI, LM of most tissues is almost fully recovered. CSF is nulled at long TI

STIR	vs	FLAIR
Short TI of 80-150 ms used.	1.	Long TI of 1500-2500 ms is used.
Combined T1 and T2 weighting is obtained	2.	Heavily T2-weighted images are obtained.
Fat, white matter can be suppressed	3.	CSF, water is suppressed
Mainly used in body imaging	4.	Used in neuroimaging
Cannot be used in post-contrast imaging as short T1 tissue are suppressed and contrast shortens T1 of tissues taking up contrast.	5.	Can be used in post-contrast imaging.

52 MRI MADE EASY (FOR BEGINNERS)

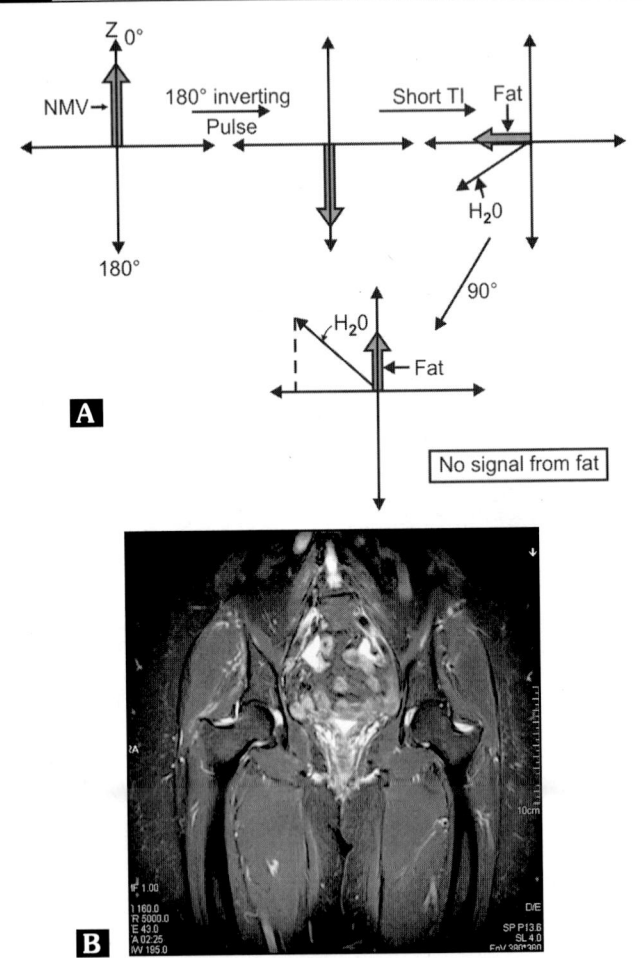

Figs 4.7A and B: STIR sequence

A. When excitatory 90° pulse is applied after short TI the magnetic vector of fat reaches zero degrees (along positive side of Z-axis). As the signal cannot be detected when the vector is vertical along Z-axis, there is no signal from fat and fat is saturated
B. STIR coronal image of the pelvis: note there is suppression of subcutaneous fat

SEQUENCES I: BASIC PRINCIPLES 53

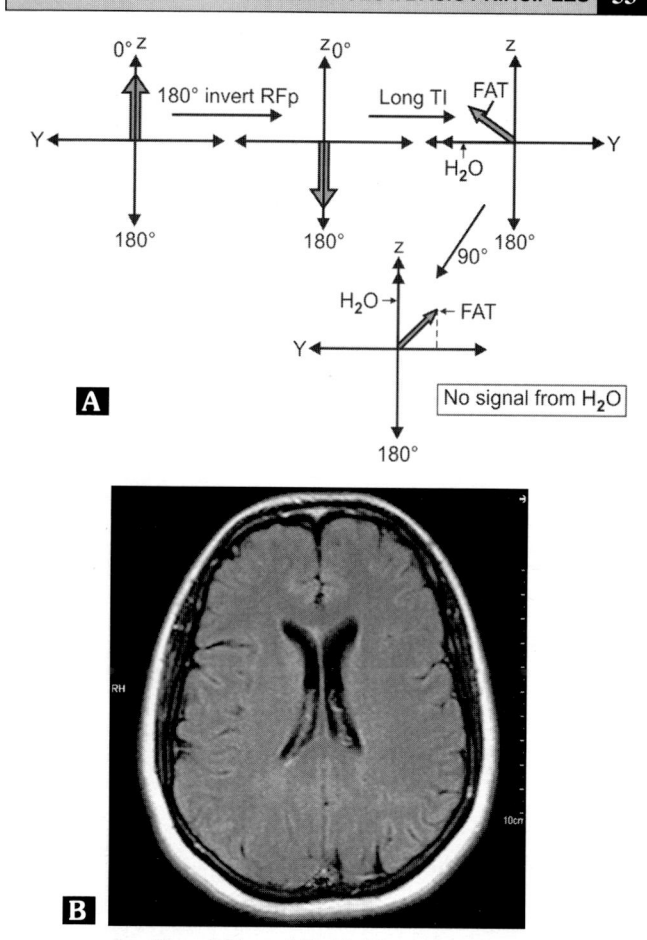

Figs 4.8A and B: FLAIR sequence

A. Magnetization vector of water reaches zero degree when 90^0 pulse is applied after long TI. Hence no signal is received from water and it is nulled
B. FLAIR axial image of brain: CSF is suppressed and is dark. Note scalp fat is not suppressed and is bright

since water has long T1. With CSF nulling in Flair, long TEs can be used to get heavily T2-wieghted without problem from CSF partial volume effects and artefacts. As in STIR, most of the pathologies appear bright on FLAIR.

GRADIENT ECHO SEQUENCE (GRE)

There are basic three differences between SE and GRE sequences.

1. There is no 180 degree pulse in GRE. Rephasing of TM in GRE is done by gradients; particularly by reversal of frequency encoding gradient. Since rephasing by gradient gives signal this sequence is called as Gradient echo sequence.
2. Flip angle in GRE are smaller, usually less than 90 degree. Since flip angle is smaller there will be early recovery of LM such that TR can be reduced hence scanning time.
3. Transverse relaxation in SE sequence is caused by combination of two mechanisms-
   A. Irreversible dephasing of TM resulting from nuclear, molecular and macromolecular magnetic interactions with proton.
   B. Dephasing caused by magnetic field inhomogeneity.

In SE sequence the dephasing caused by inhomogeneity is eliminated by 180 degree pulse. Hence there is 'true' relaxation in SE sequence. In GRE sequence dephasing effects of magnetic field inhomogeneity are not compensated as there is no 180 degree pulse. T2 relaxation in GRE is called as T2* (T2 star) relaxation.

$1/T2* = 1/T2 + 1/$ relaxation by inhomogeneity

Usually T2* < T2.

So, basic or conventional GRE sequence is as shown in the diagram (Fig. 4.9).

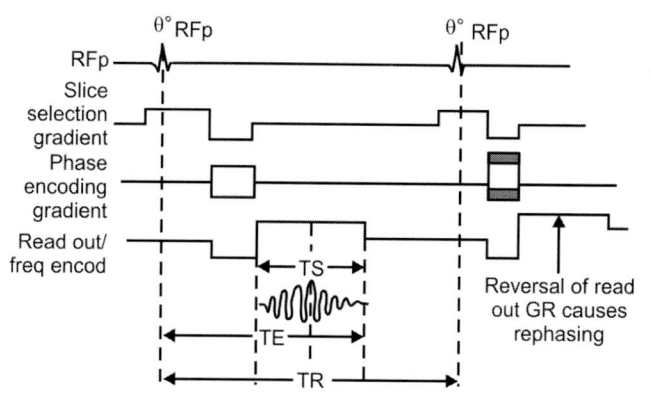

Fig. 4.9: Gradient echo sequence (GRE). Reversal of frequency encoding gradient (instead of 180 pulse) causes rephasing of protons after RFp is switched off

THE STEADY STATE (SS)

The steady state is a state in which not only LM and TM are present at the same time but also their value or magnitude is maintained steady during data acquisition.

How is steady state achieved?

Steady state is achieved by keeping TR shorter than T1 and T2 times of tissues (Fig. 4.10). Since TR is shorter than T2 there is no time for TM to decay completely, before

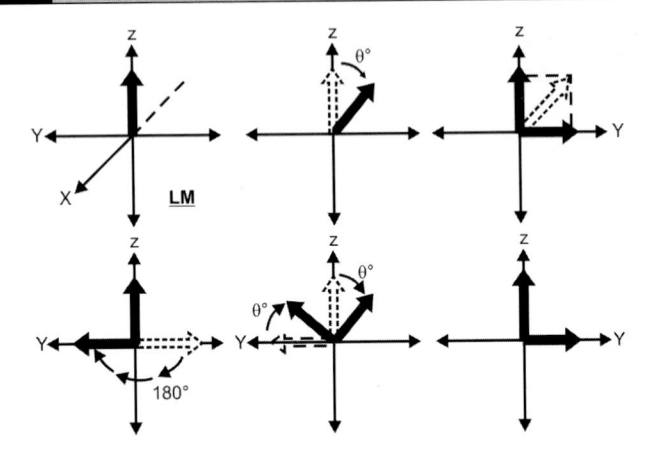

Fig. 4.10: Steady state

next RF pulse excitation. So, there will be some residual TM left over. Second factor contributing for SS is low flip angle usually 30-45 degree. Since NMV is flipped by less than 90 degrees there is always some residual LM left.

How magnitudes of LM and TM are maintained steady?
Residual TM is flipped by gradients through 180 degree from along positive side of Y-axis to negative side of Y-axis. When next RF excitation is done this residual TM along negative side of Y-axis is moved towards Z-axis. This adds up into magnitude of residual LM, which now increases. At the same time some part of the residual LM is flipped by same flip angle so that TM is formed along the positive side of Y-axis. This cycle is repeated with every RF excitation and values of LM and TM are maintained.

Why do we want steady state?

With steady state shortest TR and scan time are achieved. It also affects image contrast as it causes tissues with long T2 appear more bright on the image.

Types of Steady State

Depending on what is done to residual TM after gradient echo is received, SS can be of three types-

1. Coherent (in-phase) residual TM
   Uses variable flip angle excitation pulses followed by gradient repahsing. Since residual TM is rephased by gradients and it is in phase, it is called as coherent residual TM. Both LM and TM are maintained steady.
   Examples—FISP, GRASS

2. Incoherent (spoiled) residual TM
   In this residual TM after gradient echo is obtained is **spoiled or dephased** so that its effect on image contrast is minimal. Spoiling can be done by RF pulses or gradients. This is not classically a steady-state sequence as only LM is maintained steady and TM is spoiled.
   Examples—FLASH sequence in which residual TM is spoiled by gradients.

3. Steady state free precession (SSFP)
   Any RF pulse contains radio waves of different amplitudes. For example 90 degree RF pulse may have few 10, 70, 60, 180 or other degree radio waves such that average amplitude of RF pulse will be 90 degree.

58 MRI MADE EASY (FOR BEGINNERS)

180 degree radio waves present in the next RF pulse causes rephasing of residual TM of previous RF pulse in SSFP. Shortest possible TR and scan time can be achieved with SSFP. It is used to acquire images with true T2 weighting (since 180 degree waves used to rephase). 2D and 3D imaging is possible.

Example: PSIF.

ULTRAFAST SEQUENCES

Rapid scanning techniques are either based on low flip angle with gradient reversal or on RF refocusing. Low flip angle with gradient reversal reduces TR hence the scanning time. By using multiple refocusing RF pulses multiple lines of k-space are filled every TR thus making the acquisition rapid.

Ultrafast scanning techniques can be SE, GRE or combination of both. Major ultrafast scanning techniques include RARE, STEAM (SE) and subsecond FLASH and EPI (GRE).

Single shot RARE: (rapid acquisition with relaxation enhancement)

RARE is fast spin-echo sequence, which is nowadays called as Turbo SE or Fast SE. All the Fourier lines are filled in single sweep or single TR. RARE is a heavily T2-weighted sequence with TE in the range of 900. Therefore, it provides sufficient signal intensities only for those component that exhibit very long T2 relaxation time like fluids. RARE shows body liquids with character of angiography and is used to obtain MR cholangiogram, MR myelogram, MR urogram. Background soft tissues are not visualised in RARE.

SEQUENCES I: BASIC PRINCIPLES

High speed STEAM: (Stimulated echo acquisition method)
Any one RF pulse gives FID, any two RF pulses give spin echo and three RF pulses give stimulated echo. In STEAM three 90 degree RF pulses are used. In high speed STEAM, the final 90 degree pulse is replaced by a series of low flip angle RF pulses. Each of these low flip angle read RF pulses forms a stimulated echo, filling one line of k-space. Thus multiple k- space lines are filled in short time and in single TR.

STEAM is used in cardiac imaging, where signal from flowing blood is eliminated by dephasing of the spins. STEAM-EPI can be combined to acquire diffusion weighted images. The most important application of STEAM is in MR spectroscopy.

Subsecond FLASH (fast low angle shot)
Subsecond FLASH is possible because of availability of high gradient strengths of more than 25 mT/m. With this gradient strength TRs of 2-5 ms and TEs of 1-3 ms are easily achieved so that k-space can be filled very fast with one gradient echo per TR. Unlike FLASH, in subsecond FLASH data is acquired before a steady state is reached. $T2^*$ dephasing effects are also less because of this acquisition speed.

Subsecond FLASH can be used in body imaging where physiological motion needs to be overcome, e.g. peristaltic motions. It is also used in cardiac perfusion and combined with presaturation IR pulse to null blood signals.

EPI: Echo Plannar Imaging

Scanning time can be reduced by filling multiple lines of k-space in single TR. EPI takes this concept to extreme and all the lines of k-space are filled in a single TR. So image is formed in single TR in EPI. Since entire 2D raw data set (i.e. a plane of data or echo) could be filled during a single echo decay, the term 'Echo Plannar Imaging' was given to this technique by Sir Peter Mansfield in 1977.

Multiple echoes are generated in single TR in EPI and each is phase encoded by a different slope of gradient to fill all the required lines of k-space. These multiple echoes are either generated by 180 degree rephasing pulses or by gradient. Therefore, EPI can be Spin Echo EPI (SE-EPI) or Gradient echo EPI (GRE-EPI). However, in SE-EPI multiple 180 degree RF pulses cause excessive energy deposition in patient tissues and long train of 180 degree pulses would take so long time that most of the signal would be lost before satisfactory data could be acquired. Hence SE-EPI is not routinely used.

In GRE-EPI, rephasing is done by rapidly switching read out and phase encoding gradients on and off. This requires gradients with higher strength more than 20 mT/m.

GRE-EPI is very sensitive to susceptibility artifacts because $T2^*$ decay is not compensated in GRE sequences. Also SNR is poor in single shot EPI. To overcome these problems hybrid sequences have been devised. Hybrid sequence combines gradient and RF pulses to get advantages- the speed (gradients) and compensation of $T2^*$ effects (RF pulses). To improve SNR multi-shot EPI is used. In multishot EPI segmented scanning of k-space

SEQUENCES I: BASIC PRINCIPLES

is done by filling a portion of k-space per TR. Multi-shot EPI improves SNR and spatial resolution, gives better PD and T1-weighting at the cost of slight increase in time.

Applications of EPI:

EPI has revolutionised MR imaging with its speed. EPI has potential of interventional and real time MRI. Presently, it is used in:

1. EPI diffusion imaging
2. EPI perfusion imaging
3. Functional imaging with BOLD
4. Echo planar cardiac imaging
5. Abdominal imaging

FEW OTHER CONSIDERATIONS

Apart from basic RF pulses and gradients, certain things can be added or changed in a sequence to get specific information or improve the image. These additions or manipulations can be to improve contrast, to suppress signal from certain tissues or to reduce artifacts.

1. Preparatory and concluding pulses

   Preparatory pulse precedes the main pulse. Preparatory pulse can be used to improve contrast (e.g. MPRAGE), to supress certain tissues (e.g. fat suppression in STIR) or to reduce artifacts. Concluding pulse included at the end of the pulse sequence (Fig. 4.11).

2. Manipulations of echo or images

   Images or echoes can be combined to get new sequence. For example, images with different T2-

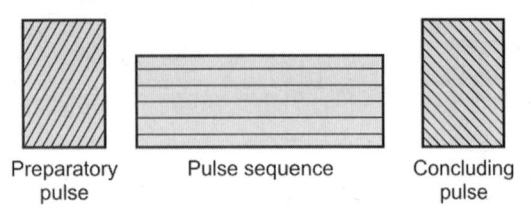

Fig. 4.11: Block diagram of sequences

weighting combined to get MEDIC sequence. Images from FISP and PSIF sequences are combined to get DESS sequence.

3. Schemes in k-space manipulations
   A. iPAT (integrated parallel acquisition technique)
      In this technique image data acquisition is done simultaneously by two or more receiver coils with different spatial sensitivities. This reduces time by half.
   B. Interpolation technique
   C. Elliptical scanning of k-space making sequence faster
   D. Key hole imaging
      Only for first image k-space is completely filled. On subsequent images only central (approximately 20%) is filled. Rest 80% is filled from first image. This results in significant reduction of scanning time. Mainly used in contrast enhanced MR angiography (Fig. 4.12).
   E. Segmented scanning of k-space fills k-space in parts
   F. Partial Fourier
      Only part of k-space is filled. Rest is calculated from its symmetry, e.g. HASTE sequence.

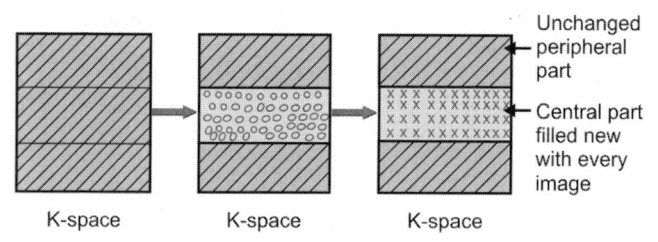

Fig. 4.12: Key-hole imaging

4. Artifact reducing techniques
   A. PACE (Perspective Acquisition Correction)
      Diaphragmatic gating done with navigator placed on diaphragm with one-half on liver and other on lung.
   B. IPAT
      Reduces motion artifacts
   C. Flow compensation
      Gradient motion rephasing corrects phase shift caused by motion
   D. LOTA (long-term averaging technique)
      Reduces breathing, motion artifacts by averaging two or more complete k-spaces as against normal averaging where each line in k-space is averaged individually.
   E. ROPE (respiratory ordered phase encoding technique)
      Reduces respiratory artifacts.
   F. ECG triggering
      Synchronises acquisitions with particular phase of cardiac cycle

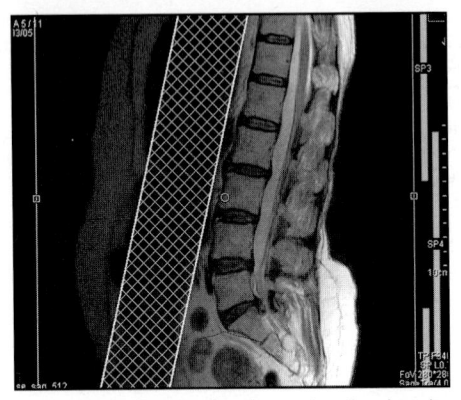

Fig. 4.13: Image showing saturation band anterior to the spine

G. Saturation band

Reduces artifacts from adjacent tissues by saturating them (Fig. 4.13).

5. SNR improving techniques.

TONE (Tilt optimized non-saturated excitation): Utilises varying flip angle in an MR angiography sequences so that saturation effect is gradual and there is no loss of signal due to saturation effect. Distal parts of vessels are well-visualized with this technique.

MTC (magnetisation transfer contrast): reduces visible MR signal from specific 'semi-solid' tissue resulting into increased contrast to noise ratio with fluid component. Useful in MR angiography and muscle studies.

SEQUENCES I: BASIC PRINCIPLES

Table 4.1: Summary of sequences

Sequence	Siemens*	GE*	Philips*
1. **Spin Echo sequence**			
Conventional SE (90-180 RF pulses)	SE	SE	SE
Double SE (90 followed by two 180 RF pulses)	PD/T2		
Multi SE (90 followed by multiple 180 RF pulses)	Turbo SE	Fast SE	Turbo SE
Single shot Multi SE (Multi SE with half k-space filling)	HASTE	Single shot FSE	Ultrafast SE
2. **Inversion Recovery Sequence**			
Short TI (80-150 ms) e.g. STIR			
Medium TI (200-800 ms) e.g. MPRAGE			
Long TI (1500-2500 ms) e.g. FLAIR			
3. **Gradient Echo Sequence**			
A. Incoherent spoiled TM	FLASH	SPGR	T1-FFE
B. Coherent/Rephased TM			
1. Post excitation refocused (FID sampled)	FISP	GRASS	FFE
2. Pre-excitation refocused (Spin echo sampled)	PSIF	SSFP	T2-FFE
3. Fully refocused (both FID and spin echo sampled)	True FISP	FIESTA	Balanced FFE
4. **Hybrid**			
Combination of SE and GRE	TGSE	GRASE	GRASE
5. **EPI**			
Single shot			
Multishot-segmented			

*Vendor nomenclatures for sequences are taken from References- 1. Nitz WR. MR Imaging: Acronyms and clinical applications. Eur Radiol. 1999;9:979-997. and 2. Brown MA, Semelka RC. MR Imaging Abbreviations, Definitions, and Descriptions: A Review. Radiology 1999; 213:647-662.

CHAPTER 5

Sequences II: Few Common Sequences

68 MRI MADE EASY (FOR BEGINNERS)

INTRODUCTION

In this chapter few commonly used sequences, other than T1 and T2-weighted images, in routine practice will be discussed. Basic type of the sequence and its uses with illustrations are explained. See Figure 5.1 for parameters on the image.

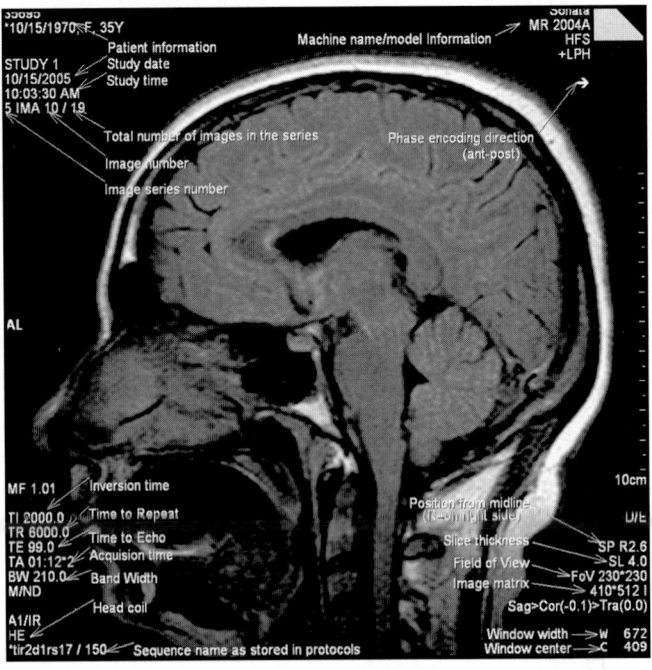

Fig. 5.1: Image parameters

1. FLASH

Fast Low Angle Shot.

Type: Gradient Echo

Spoiled (incoherent) residual transverse magnetization.

SEQUENCES II: FEW COMMON SEQUENCES

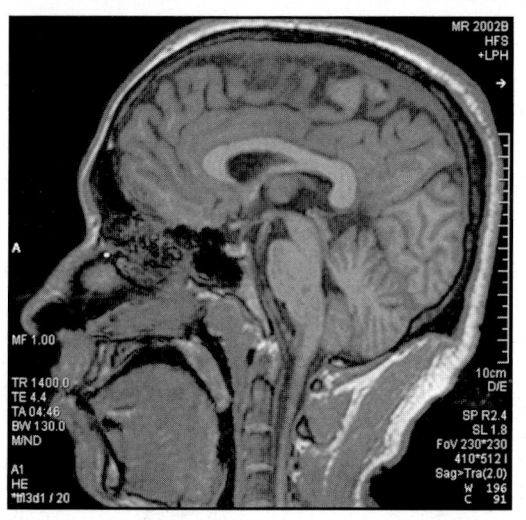

Fig. 5.2: T1-weighted FLASH sagittal image of normal brain

FLASH (Siemens) is similar to SPGR (GE).

Uses:
1. In brain imaging high resolution T1-weighted 3D acquisition can be done pre and post contrast (Fig. 5.2).
2. T2-weighted FLASH images show acute bleed as dark signal and is very useful to detect cerebral haemorrhage (Fig. 5.3).
3. Flow and angiographic studies can be performed with FLASH.
4. Cardiac Imaging: FLASH is useful in visualisation of cardiac motion, wall thickness and valves accomplished by ECG synchronisation.
5. Dynamic scanning for physiological motions and contrast enhancement: First phase of susceptibility

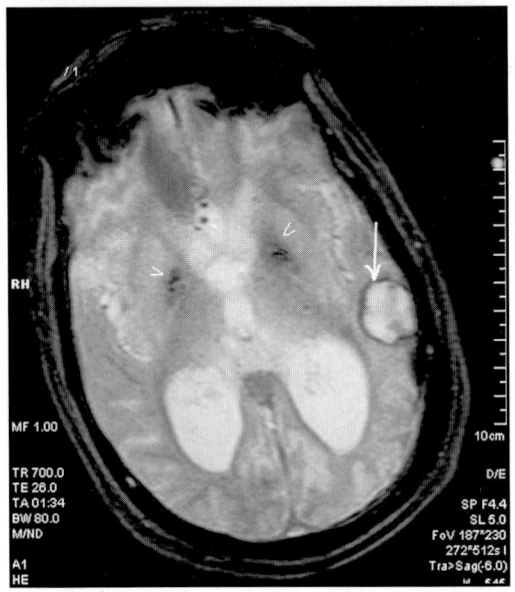

Fig. 5.3: Gradient Hemo axial image of brain. Hemorrhage—dark rim (arrow) is noted in the left temporo-occipital region. Bilateral basal ganglion calcifications also noted (arrowheads)

induced signal loss (T2* contrast) is used in MR perfusion. Second phase of decreased T1 causing high signal is used in assessing tumor vascularity in MR Mammography (Fig. 5.4).

6. FLASH can be used in functional brain mapping by BOLD (blood oxygen level dependent) imaging.

2. FLAIR

Fluid Attenuated Inversion Recovery.

SEQUENCES II: FEW COMMON SEQUENCES 71

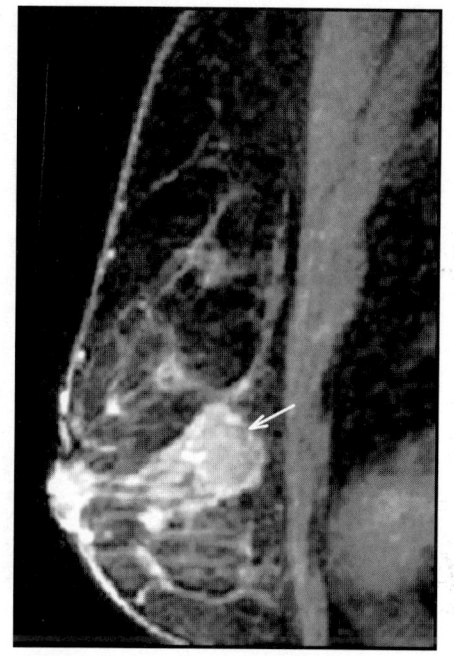

Fig. 5.4: FLASH sagittal image of the breast shows an enhancing lesion (arrows)

Type: Inversion Recovery. Long TI (1500-2500 ms). CSF is effectively suppressed. Thus heavily T2-weighted images can be obtained without problems from CSF partial volume effects and artifacts.

Uses

Flair is used in neuroimaging.

1. Extent of perilesional edema can be determined easily (Fig. 5.5).
2. Brain infarctions are well seen on Flair (Fig. 5.6).

72 MRI MADE EASY (FOR BEGINNERS)

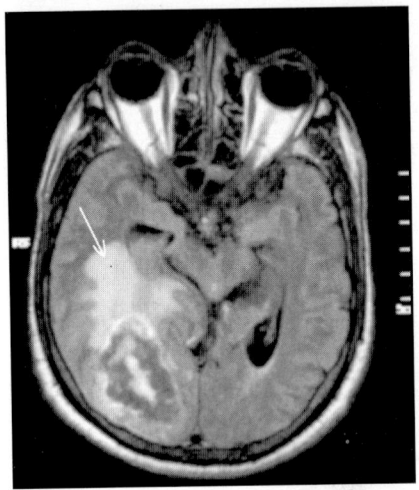

Fig. 5.5: FLAIR axial image of the brain showing a large tumor in right hemisphere. Note the edema anterior to the lesion (arrow).

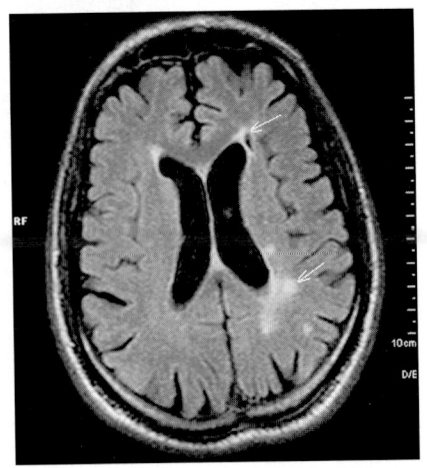

Fig. 5.6: FLAIR axial image of the brain. Note multiple chronic infarcts in left periventricular region indicated by arrows

SEQUENCES II: FEW COMMON SEQUENCES

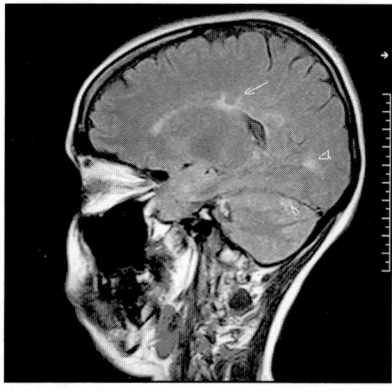

Fig. 5.7: FLAIR sagittal image of the brain. Multiple plaques are seen running perpendicular to the callosal margin (arrow) called as 'Dowson's fingers'. Also seen are plaques in the occipital lobe and the cerebellum (arrowheads).

3. Bright lesions of multiple sclerosis better seen on FLAIR (Fig. 5.7).
4. Increased signal in mesial temporal sclerosis is better appreciated on FLAIR (Fig. 5.8).

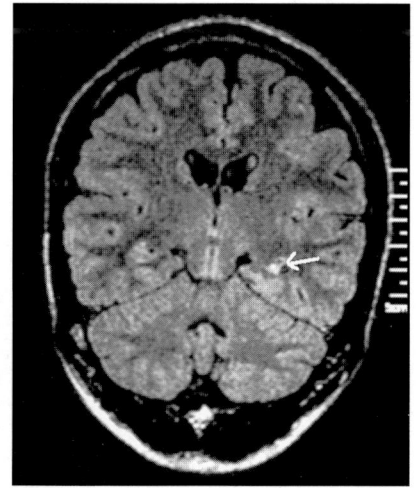

Fig. 5.8: FLAIR oblique coronal image of the brain showing hippocampi in cross-section. Bilateral hippocampi show increased signals. The left hippocampus is atrophic as well (arrow)

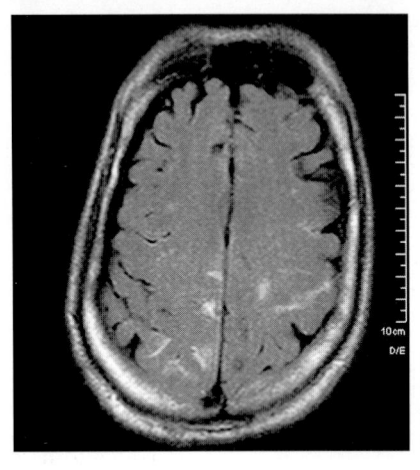

Fig. 5.9: FLAIR axial image of the brain. Bright signals suggestive of SAH are seen in cortical sulci

5. Fast FLAIR shows subarachnoid hemorrhage (Fig. 5.9).
6. Syrinx/cysts in spinal cord are well seen on FLAIR.
7. FLAIR can be used in post-contrast imaging.

3. MEDIUM TI INVERSION RECOVERY SEQUENCE

Type: Medium TI (200-800 ms) IR and Multi SE Combined

Use: Very good gray-white matter differentiation can be obtained with this sequence. It shows cortical dysplasias well. This sequence forms a part of temporal lobe epilepsy protocol (Fig. 5.10).

4. CISS

Constructive Interference at Steady State.

Type: Gradient echo. T2-weighted. 3D.

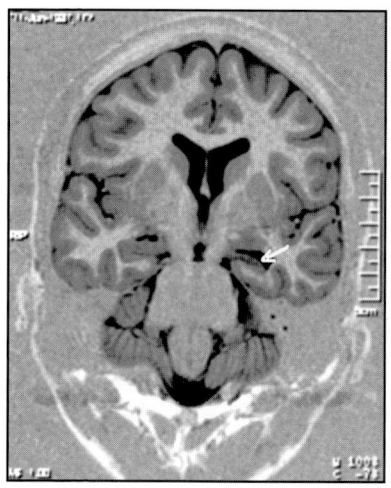

Fig. 5.10: Medium TI inversion recovery oblique coronal image of the brain shows atrophic left hippocampus (arrow). Note the white background of the image. This is because the image is inverted. Air never produces any signal on any of the sequences. It is always dark

CISS combines two true FISP images acquired separately with some modifications.

Uses: 3D acquisition of posterior cranial fossa gives high resolution images showing cranial nerves dark against background of bright CSF. CISS is routinely performed for suspected internal auditory canal and cerebello-pontine angle cistern pathologies (Fig. 5.11). CISS can also be used to visualise spinal nerve roots and optic nerve.

5. MPRAGE

Magnetization Prepared Rapid Acquisition Gradient Echo.

Type: combination of medium TI inversion recovery and gradient echo.

76 MRI MADE EASY (FOR BEGINNERS)

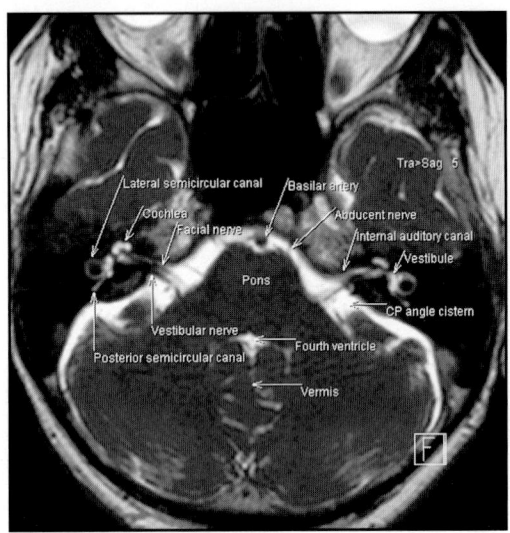

Fig. 5.11: CISS axial image of CP angle region. See the dark cranial nerves against the background of bright CSF

Uses: Thin slice 3D of the brain can be obtained. Shows good gray-white contrast and can be used instead of routine T2-weighted sequence. The sequence can also be used in post contrast imaging (Fig. 5.12).

6. STIR

Short TI Inversion Recovery.
Type: Short inversion time (TI)—80-150 ms.
    both T1 and T2 weighting to images.

Uses: Pathology stands out in STIR images and it is very easy to pick up lesions. Hence, STIR is used

SEQUENCES II: FEW COMMON SEQUENCES

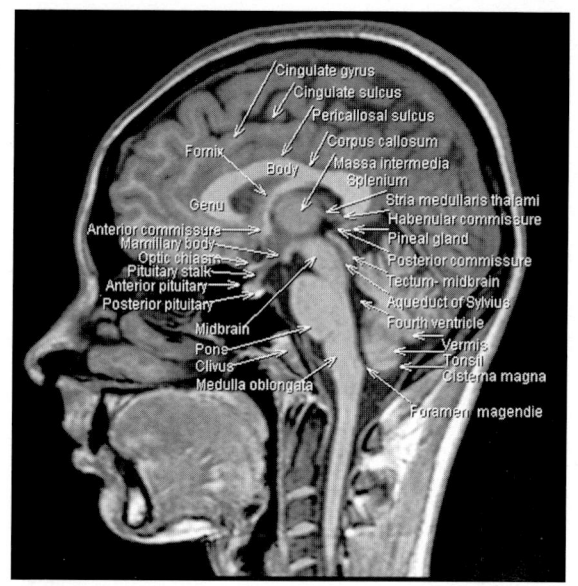

Fig. 5.12: MPRAGE sagittal image of the brain. Appreciate the gray-white differentiation ability of the sequence.

almost everywhere in the body imaging. Few common uses are:

1. Bone marrow imaging: STIR shows marrow edema very well. It is very useful detecting multiple lesions in bones and now used for bone metastases screening (Figs 5.13 and 5.14).
2. It is used orbital imaging specially for optic nerves (Fig. 5.15).
3. It is used in SI joint imaging and shows marrow edema earlier than erosions seen on CT scan in arthropathies (Fig. 5.16).

78 MRI MADE EASY (FOR BEGINNERS)

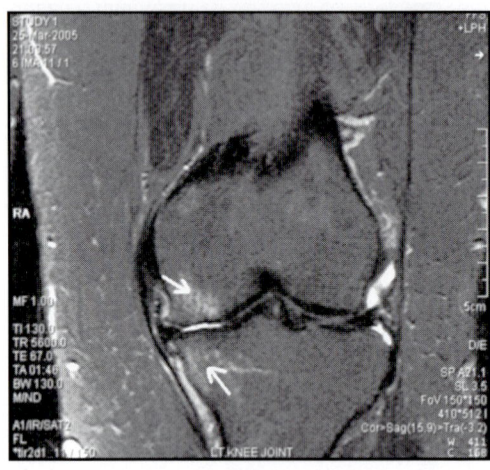

Fig. 5.13: STIR coronal image of the knee. Bright signals are seen in medial condyles of tibia and femur (arrow) suggestive of marrow edema

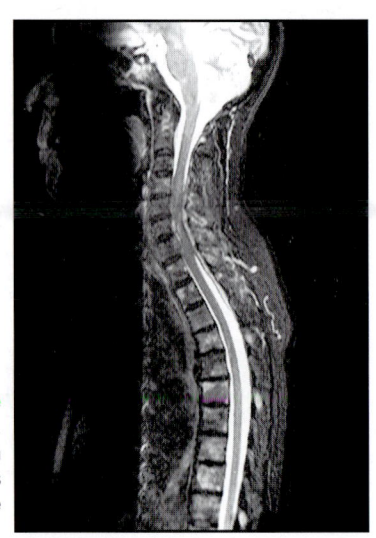

Fig. 5.14: STIR sagittal image of the cervicodorsal spine. Multiple bright spots are seen in vertebral bodies as well as posterior elements suggestive of metastases

SEQUENCES II: FEW COMMON SEQUENCES 79

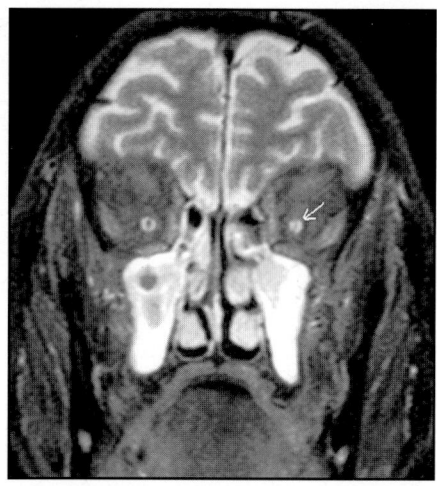

Fig. 5.15: STIR coronal image of the orbit. The left optic nerve is atrophic with prominent CSF space around it (arrow)

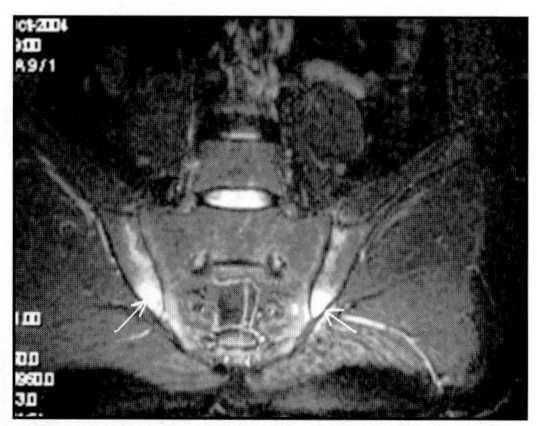

Fig. 5.16: STIR axial image of sacroiliac joints in ankylosing spondylitis. Early inflammatory changes in the form of edema are seen as bright signals bilaterally (arrows)

7. TRUFI

True FISP: Free Induction at Steady State
Type: Gradient echo.

Steady state with rephased (coherent) residual transverse magnetization.

True FISP combines echoes from FISP and PSIF (SSFP) to have very fast T2-weighted images. FISP (Siemens) is similar to GRASS (GE).

Uses:

Rapid breath-hold scanning can be obtained with trufi. Hence, it is very useful and commonly used in-
1. Abdominal imaging (Fig. 5.17)
2. Cardiac imaging (Fig. 5.18)
3. Fetal imaging (Fig. 5.19)
4. MR enteroclysis.

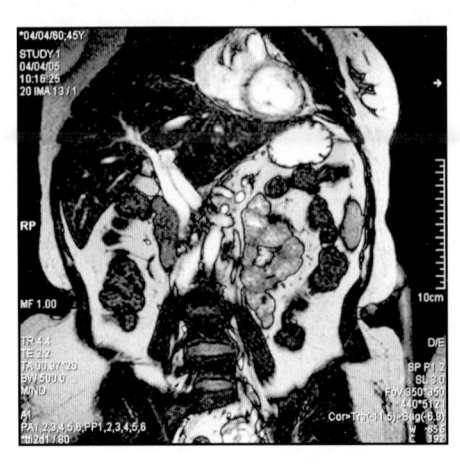

Fig. 5.17: True FISP coronal image of the abdomen in a normal patient. Note the bright vessels and biliary ducts

SEQUENCES II: FEW COMMON SEQUENCES 81

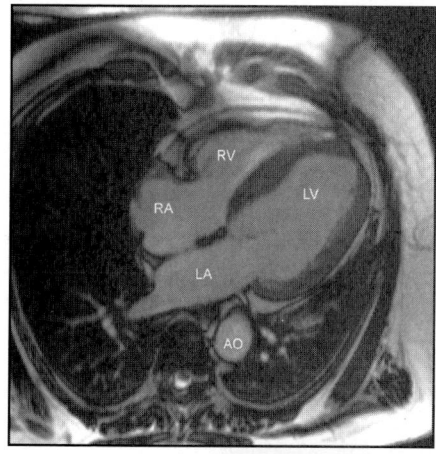

Fig. 5.18: True FISP four chamber view of the normal heart. Myocardium and valves are seen as dark signal against bright blood in the chamber. LA- left atrium, LV-left vetricle, RA-right atrium, RV- right ventricle

Fig. 5.19: True FISP image of the gravid uterus. Appreciate the head of the fetus (arrow), liver (arrowhead), urinary bladder (UB) and uterine wall (UW)

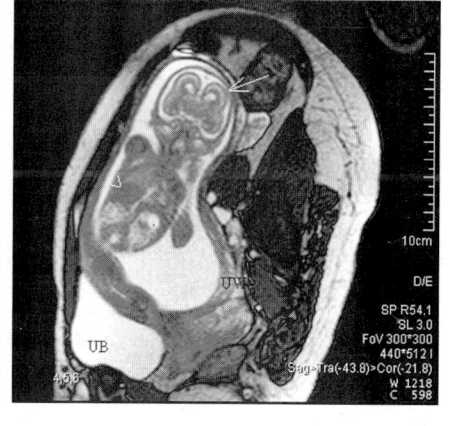

8. HASTE

Half Fourier Acquisition with Turbo Spin Echo.

Type: Turbo spin echo.

Partial Fourier—only half the k-space is filled to reduce scan time.

82 MRI MADE EASY (FOR BEGINNERS)

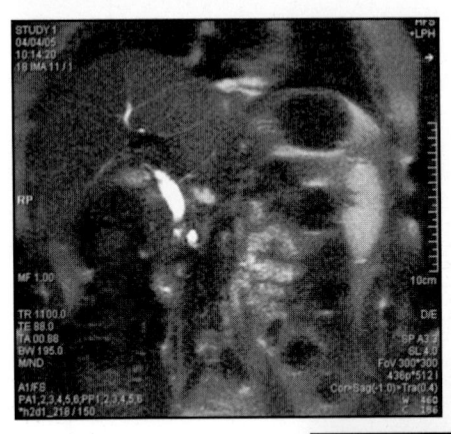

Fig. 5.20: HASTE coronal image of the normal abdomen. Note slight haziness of the image. This is because loss of signal due to T2 decay

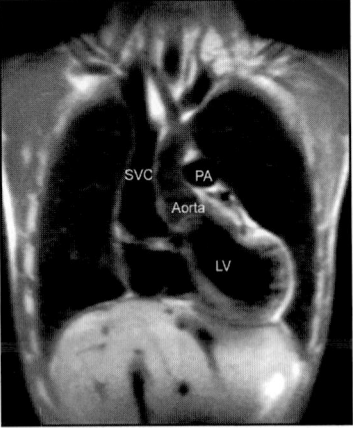

Fig. 5.21: HASTE coronal image of the heart. HASTE is a spin-echo sequence hence blood in the vessels and chamber is dark. PA-pulmonary artery, LV- left ventricle, SVC- superior vena cava

Uses: Apart from MRCP, HASTE is useful in:
1. Abdominal imaging (Fig. 5.20).
2. Cardiac imaging (Fig. 5.21).
3. MR myelogram (Fig. 5.22).
4. MR enteroclysis (Fig. 5.23).

SEQUENCES II: FEW COMMON SEQUENCES 83

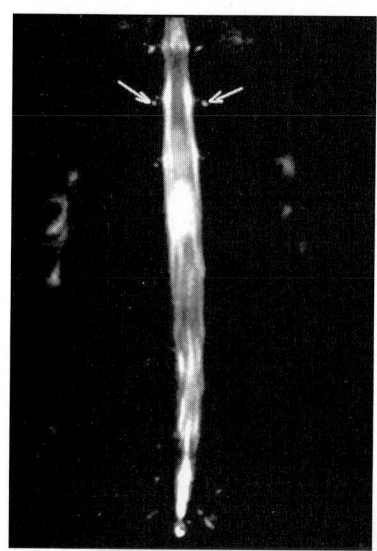

Fig. 5.22: MR Myelogram: This HASTE coronal image. Arrows indicate nerve roots. The background tissues are suppressed because of the very high TE in the range of 1100-1200 ms

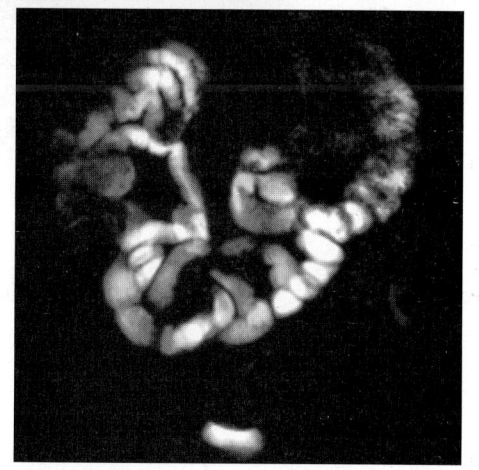

Fig. 5.23: MR enteroclysis. Bowel loops are seen as white loops in this HASTE coronal image

9. DESS

Double echo in Steady State.

Type: Gradient echo. Steady state.

DESS combines two images from (as against Trufi, which combines echoes) FISP and PSIF. DESS has both T1 and T2 contrast hence anatomy as well as fluid are seen very well.

Uses: DESS with water excitation pre-pulse is used in joint imaging, where it shows articular cartilage, bone and synovial fluid very well. Data can be post processed using MIP and MPR (Fig. 5.24).

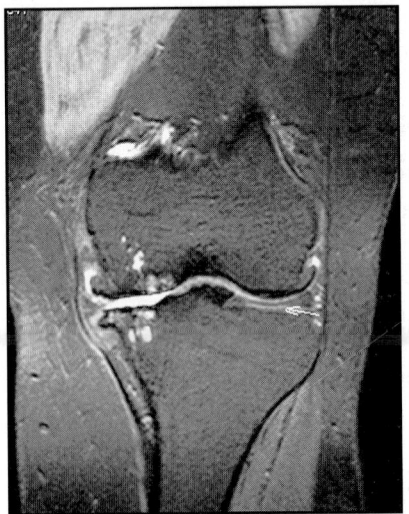

Fig. 5.24: DESS coronal image of the knee. Medial compartment osteoarthritis is seen with subchondral (bright) cysts and osteophytes. Note the normal articular cartilage (arrow) in the lateral compartment seen as moderately high intensity structure

SEQUENCES II: FEW COMMON SEQUENCES

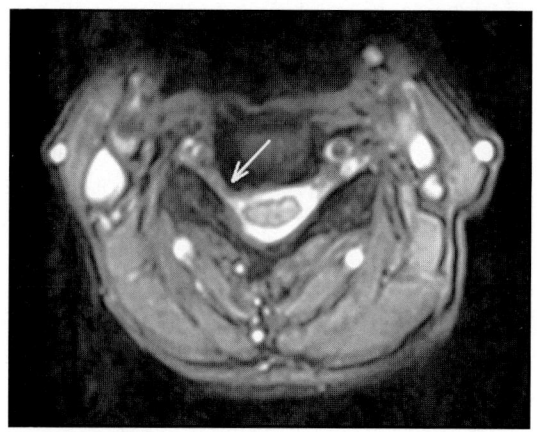

Fig. 5.25: MEDIC axial image of the cervical spine. Right posterolateral disc herniation is seen as dark structure (arrow) encroaching on the neural foramen

10. MEDIC

Multi Echo Data Image Combination
Type: Gradient echo. RF spoiled.

Medic combines images with different T2-weighting.

Has minimal flow artifacts and less sensitivity to susceptibility and chemical shift effects

Uses: Used in cervical spine imaging with flow compensation to avoid artifacts from neck vessels (Fig. 5.25).

11. VIBE

Volume Interpolated Breath-hold Imaging
Type: 3D FLASH with volume interpolation.

Gradient echo. RF spoiling+.

Short TR/TE with low flip angle. Rapid acquisitions.

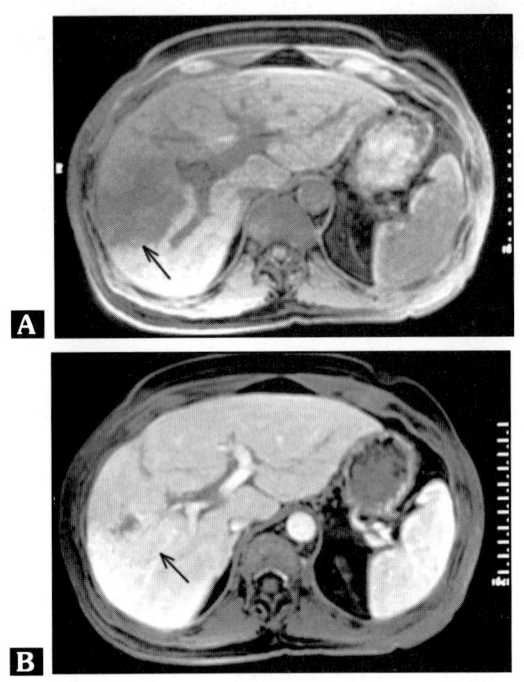

Figs 5.26A and B: VIBE axial images of abdomen. (A) Precontrast image shows a liver lesion (arrow), which enhances on post-contrast image (B)

Uses: This rapid sequence can be used in pre and post contrast body imaging since acquisitions can be done in breath-holds. Useful in post-contrast multiphase studies (Figs 5.26A and B).

CHAPTER 6

Artifacts

INTRODUCTION

MR imaging also suffers from artifacts as other radiological modalities. Artifacts can cause significant image degradation and can lead to misinterpretation. It is impossible to eliminate all artifacts though they can be reduced to acceptable level. With newer techniques coming up newer artifacts are added. In this chapter we will discuss few common artifacts, their causes and measures to reduce them. Artifacts occur along particular axis of gradient hence axis along which the artifact occurs is given with each artifact.

GHOSTS

Ghosts are replica of something in the image. Ghosts are produced by anatomy moving along a gradient during pulse sequence resulting into phase mismapping. Ghosts can originate from any structure that moves during the acquisition of data (Fig. 6.1).

Axis

Ghosts always occur along phase encoding axis.

Causes

Motion is the most important cause of ghost artifacts. Ghosts can also be caused by mechanical vibration, temporal variation of receiver coil sensitivity, fluctuations of magnetic field, imbalance of quadrature channels and stimulated echoes.

ARTIFACTS 89

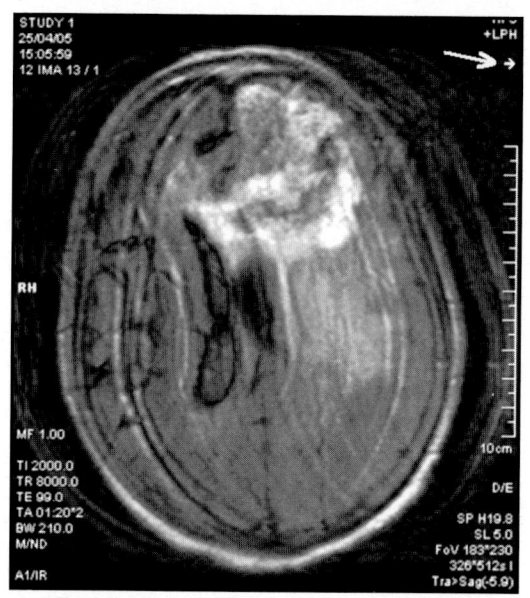

Fig. 6.1: Ghosting-Movement artifacts. Note the phase encoding direction (right to left) indicated by the arrow

Corrective Measures

1. Phase encoding axis swap: Phase encoding direction is changed.
   For example—In sagittal image of the spine with phase encoding along y-axis (anterior to posterior) pulsatile motion of aorta causes ghosting over the spinal cord. If phase encoding gradient is applied along Z-axis (head to foot) this artifact will not overlap over the spinal cord.

2. **Presaturation**—Area producing motion artifacts is saturated with RF pulses before start of proper pulse sequence such that all signals from this area are eliminated.

   For example—In sagittal image of the cervical spine swallowing produces ghosts along phase axis (anterior-posterior) and obscures the spinal cord. To eliminate this presaturation pulses are applied anterior to the cervical spine over esophagus.

3. **Ordered phase encoding**—Center of k-space is responsible for SNR and is filled with shallow phase encoding gradient slope. Shallow slope of phase encoding gradient results in good signal amplitude. When gradient slope is shallow the phase shift caused by movement is less resulting in less ghosting. In ordered phase encoding, which is applied in regular periodic movement, center of k-space is filled when movement is minimum so that less ghosting and good SNR is achieved. Periphery of k-space is filled with steep slope of phase encoding gradient when movement is maximum.

   For example—Respiratory ordered phase encoding (ROPE) (Fig. 6.2). When motion of the chest wall is maximum, i.e. inspiration, steep slopes of phase encoding gradients are applied. When motion of the chest wall is minimum, i.e. expiration shallow phase encoding gradient slopes are applied.

4. **Gating**—ECG, pulse or respiratory gating.

   Data acquisition is done in particular phase of cardiac or respiratory cycle in every cycle.

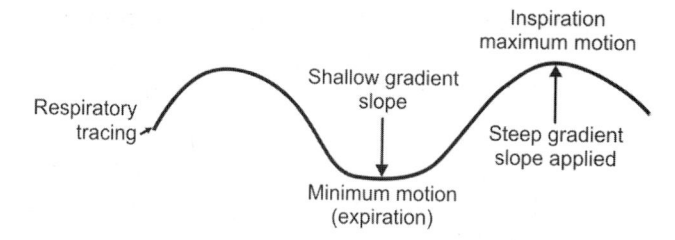

Fig. 6.2: Respiratory ordered phase encoding

5. Gradient moment nulling/ rephasing—Reduces ghosts caused by flowing nuclei moving along gradients by adjusting the gradient. GMR is used to reduce ghosts in gradient echo sequence.

ALIASING/ WRAPAROUND

In aliasing, anatomy that exists outside the FOV appear in an image. Anatomy outside the selected FOV produces signal if it is in close proximity to the receiver coil. During signal encoding, signals from this outside FOV structures are also allocated pixel positions. If frequencies of these signals are higher than the limit that can be sampled, these frequencies are given pixel positions within FOV on lower frequency side. Hence there is wraparound of structures outside the FOV into the image (Fig. 6.3).

Axis

Aliasing can occur along any axis. Aliasing along frequency encoding axis is called frequency wrap and along phase encoding axis is called phase wrap.

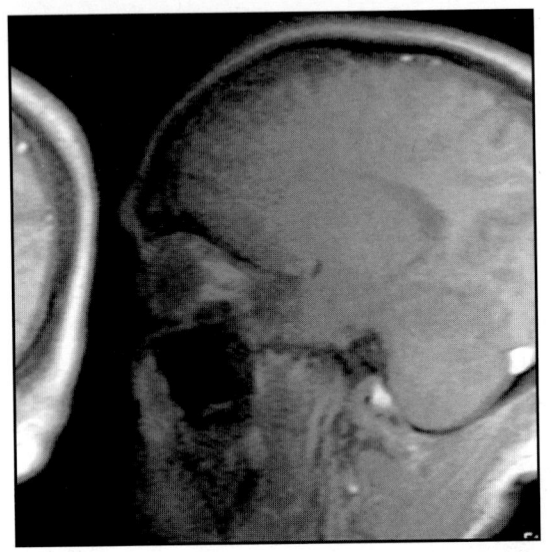

Fig. 6.3: Aliasing artifact: This FLASH sagittal image of the brain shows posterior part wrapped around and seen anteriorly

Corrective Measures

Frequency wrap—Frequency wrap is easier to correct. Low pass-filters are used to cut-off the frequencies originating from outside FOV.

Phase wrap—Phase wrap can be corrected by increasing FOV along phase encoding direction. However, increasing FOV causes reduction in spatial resolution.

CHEMICAL SHIFT RELATED ARTIFACTS

Because of different chemical environment protons in water and fat precess at different frequencies. This difference in

ARTIFACTS 93

precessional frequencies of protons in water and fat is 'chemical shift'. It is expressed in parts per million (ppm). The frequency of water protons is about 3.5 ppm greater than that of fat protons. This chemical shift of 3.5 ppm causes water protons to precess at a frequency 220 Hz higher than that of fat proton at 1.5 tesla. Chemical shift forms the basis for MR spectroscopy. However, same chemical shift becomes source of artifacts in MR imaging.

There are two types of artifacts related to chemical shift: 1. Chemical shift misregistration artifact (Fig. 6.4) and 2. Interference from chemical shift (in-phase/out-phase) (Figs 6.5A and B). These are discussed in Table 6.1.

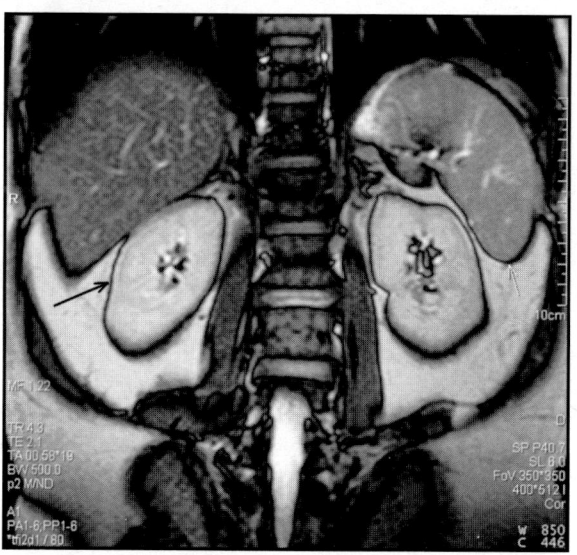

Fig. 6.4: Chemical shift misregistration artifact: Trufi coronal image of the abdomen shows dark edge around the organs specially kidneys. The susceptibility effects at tissue interface are also contributing to this dark edge

94 MRI MADE EASY (FOR BEGINNERS)

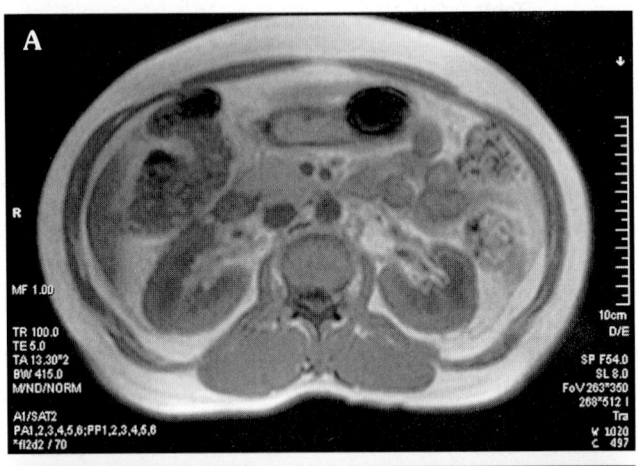

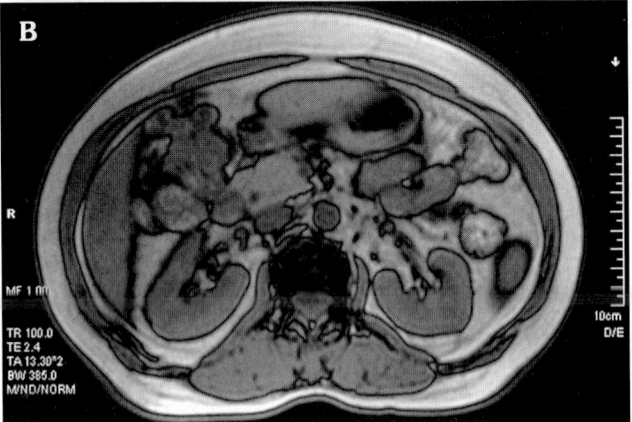

Figs 6.5A and B: In-phase image (A) at TE 5 ms, out-phase image (B) at TE 2.4 ms. Note dark edges around the kidneys

ARTIFACTS

Table 6.1: Artifacts related to chemical shift

	Chemical shift misregistration	Interference from chemical shift
1. Mechanism	Receive bandwidth is the range of frequencies that must be mapped across FOV. If bandwidth is ± 16 kHz, i.e. 32000 Hz and frequency encoding steps are 256 then each pixel has an individual frequency range of 125Hz/pixel (3200/256). At 1.5T chemical shift between water and fat is 220 Hz. Therefore, water and fat protons existing adjacent to one other are mapped 1.76 pixels apart (220/125). This pixel shift of fat relative to water results into artifacts	Since water protons precess about 220hz faster than fat protons at 1.5 T, they complete an extra revolution every 4.5 ms. So fat and water protons are in phase at certain times and out of phase at others. At TE times that are multiples of 4.5 ms at 1.5 T, they are in phase. They are out of phase at TE times halfway between the special in-phase TE times. When they are in-phase their signal add together. When out of phase their signals cancel each other out. This results in artifacts
2. Axis	Along frequency encoding axis	Phase encoding axis since caused by phase difference
3. Artifact	Dark edge at the interface between fat and water	Dark edge around certain organs where fat and water interfaces occur within same voxel
4. Corrective measures	1. Using lower field strengths since chemical shift is less and insignificant. 2. Reduce FOV. 3. Increase bandwidth.	1. Using spin-echo sequence- since 180 degree rephasing pulses compensate for phase difference between fat and water. So the artifact is reduced in SE sequence 2. Selecting TE that is multiple of 4.5 ms at 1.5 T. So that water and fat are in phase
5. Good effects	Chemical shift along frequency encoding axis forms the basis of MR spectroscopy.	In-phase and out-phase imaging is used to differentiate adrenal metastasis from adenoma

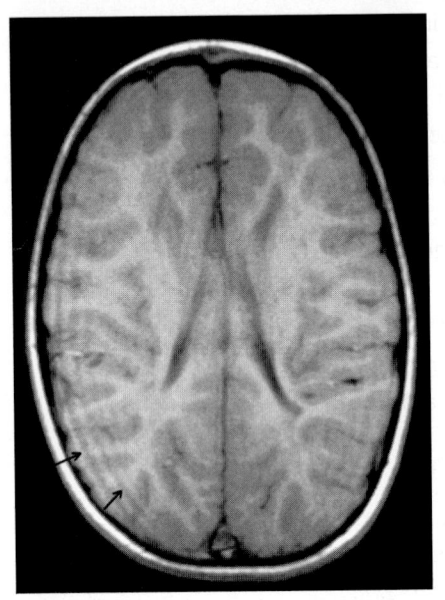

Fig. 6.6: Truncation artifacts: T1-weighted axial image of the brain shows dark linear artifacts along the periphery of the brain (arrows)

TRUNCATION ARTIFACT

Truncation artifacts are also called as edge, Gibbs' and ringing artifacts.

Truncation artifacts produce low intensity band running through high intensity area (Fig. 6.6). The artifact is caused by under sampling of the data so that interfaces of high and low signal are incorrectly represented on the image. Truncation artifacts can be misleading in long narrow structures, such as spinal cord or intervertebral disc. For

ARTIFACTS 97

example in T1-weighted sagittal image of the cervical spine CSF in central canal appears dark as compared to spinal cord and might be misinterpreted as syringomyelia. This is specifically called as Gibbs' artifact.

Axis

Phase encoding.

Corrective Measures

Increase the number of phase encoding steps.
For example—256 × 256 matrix instead of 256 × 128.

MAGNETIC SUSCEPTIBILITY ARTIFACT

Magnetic susceptibility is the ability of a substance to become magnetised. Some tissues magnetise to different degree than other, resulting into differences in precessional frequency and phase. This causes dephasing at the interface of these tissues and signal loss. For example—magnetic susceptibility difference between bone, other soft tissue and air is about 10 ppm. This causes signal loss and distortion of the boundaries of the brain near air sinuses. Other common causes of magnetic susceptibility artifacts include metal, iron content of haemorrhage.

Magnetic susceptibility is more prominent in GRE sequence than SE sequence (Fig. 6.7). In SE sequences compensation for the phase differences occurs because there is refocusing by 180 pulses of the dephasing caused by magnetic field inhomogeneities.

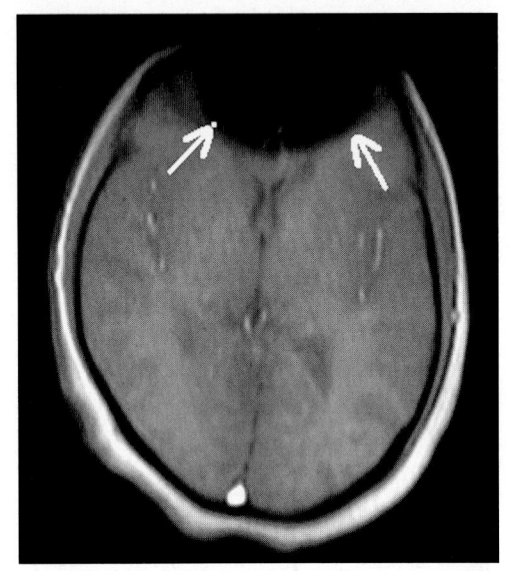

Fig. 6.7: 'Bindi artifact': This dark artifact in the axial localizer image of the brain is because of the magnetic susceptibility effect caused by some metallic components in the *bindi*.

Axis

Frequency encoding and phase encoding

Corrective Measures

1. Use of SE sequence
2. Remove all metals.

Good Effects

Magnetic susceptibility also has good effects apart from artifacts and can be useful in following ways.

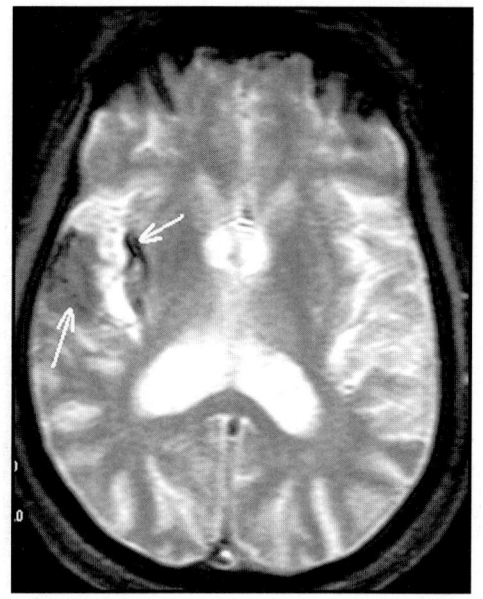

Fig. 6.8: Magnetic susceptibility effect: Gradient Hemo axial image of the brain shows bleed in the right perisylvian region (arrows)

1. Used to diagnose hemorrhage (Fig. 6.8).
2. Forms the basis of post-contrast T2*-weighted MR perfusion studies.
3. Used to quantify myocardial and liver Iron overload.

STRAIGHT LINES

Straight lines through MR images can be caused by RF interference, stimulated echo and spike in the k-space.

Radiowaves from sources outside the MR machine (from inside or outside the shielded MR room) can cause pattern of straight lines. Sources inside the room of interefaring RF could be monitoring devices or flickering light bulb.

Zipper like artifact is a line with alternating bright and dark pixels propogating along the frequency encoding direction. It is caused by stimulated echo that have missed phase encoding.

A spike in k-space causes a pattern of regularly spaced lines across an MR image (Fig. 6.9).

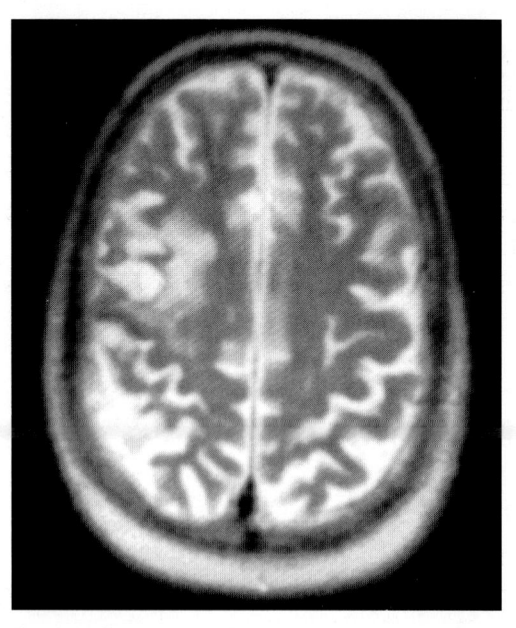

Fig. 6.9: Straight line: T2-w axial image of the brain shows straight lines throughout the image

Axis

Zipper artifact is seen along frequency encoding axis.

Corrective Measures

For RF interference site of RF leak should be located and corrected. Sources of RF inside the room should be removed. Zipper artifact can be eliminated by spoiler gradients arranged in special pattern to remove stimulated echoes.

SHADING ARTIFACTS

In shading artifact image has uneven contrast with loss of signal intensity in one part of the image (Fig. 6.10). The causes include uneven excitation of nuclei within the patient due to RF pulses applied at flip angles other than 90 and 180 degree, abnormal loading of coil or coupling of coil, inhomogeneity of magnetic field and overflow of ADC.

Axis

Frequency and phase encoding.

Corrective Measures

Load the coil correctly.

Shimming to reduce the inhomogeneity of the magnetic field.

To avoid ADC overflow, images are acquired with less amplification.

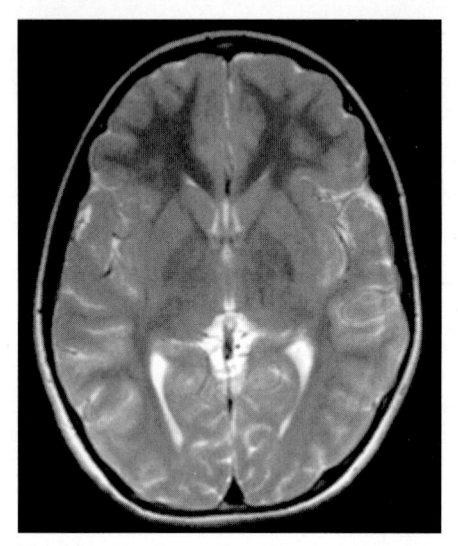

Fig. 6.10: Shading artifact: T2-w axial image of the brain shows comparatively less signal in the frontal regions. This was because of the improper loading of the coil

CROSS-EXCITATION AND CROSS-TALK

An RF excitation pulse is not exactly square. As a result nuclei in slices adjacent to the RF excitation pulse may be excited by it and receive energy. This energy flips NMV of these nuclei into transverse plane so that they are saturated when they are excited by their own RF excitation pulse. This affects contrast. This phenomenon is called *cross excitation* (Fig. 6.11).

The same effect is produced when energy is dissipated to nuclei from neighbouring slice as nuclei within the selected slice relax after RF pulse is switched off. This is called as *cross-talk*.

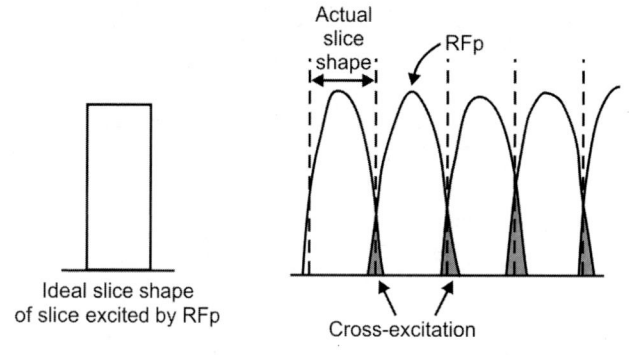

Fig. 6.11: Cross excitation

Axis

Slice selection gradient

Corrective Measures

Cross-talk cannot be corrected.
To minimise the cross-excitation:
1. Increase interslice gap.
2. Interleaved slices scanning. First slice numbers 1, 3, 5, 7 are excited and then slices 2, 4, 6, 8 are excited. So that nuclei have time to relax.

CHAPTER 7

MR Safety

INTRODUCTION

In spite of no proven hazards, MR has potentials for bio-effects. Safety precautions should be followed strictly as failure to do so can lead to life threatening incidences. This chapter is intended to make the readers aware of some potential bio-effects of MR and some safety precautions to be strictly followed to avoid any untoward effects. These safety precautions are based on recommendations in "American College of Radiology White Paper on MR Safety" published in AJR 2002;178:1335-47 and later updated in AJR 2004;182:1111-14.

Please note that safety issues discussed in this chapter are just viewpoints based on ACR white paper on MR safety and some textbooks. These are not recommendations or guidelines given by any authorised body. Therefore, author will not be responsible for any decision about scanning patients with safety issues made, based on views expressed in this chapter.

MR BIOEFFECTS

Patients undergoing MR examination is exposed to three different forms of electromagnetic radiation:
1. Static magnetic field
2. Gradient magnetic field
3. RF electromagnetic field.

Static magnetic field can raise the skin temperature. It can cause electrical induction and cardiac effects with elevation of T-wave amplitude. It also has potential effects on neurons. All these bio-effects are not proved to be hazardous at field strength below three tesla. Scanning at field strength more than three tesla has been shown to cause vertigo, headache and peripheral nerve stimulation.

Gradient field related possible effects include ventricular fibrillation, epileptogenic potentials, visual flashes. It also has thermal effects. All these effects have not been significant in presently used clinical MR systems.

RF magnetic field can result into energy deposition and tissue heating. SAR (specific absorption rate) is measure of tissue energy deposition and its unit is Watt/Kg. FDA limit for clinical examination is SAR < 0.4 W/Kg. However, no clinically hazardous effects or increased skin and body temperature were seen with SAR upto 4W/Kg in experiments. Testes and eyes are more temperature-sensitive organs.

Acoustic Noise

It is caused by vibrations of gradient coils. Noise increases with heavy duty cycles and sharper pulse transition. Noise also increases with thin slices, small FOV, less TR and TE. Ear plugs, ear phones should be provided to patients and the person accompanying.

SAFETY-RELATED ISSUES

Site Access Restriction

ACR white paper recommends that MR site should be divided into four zones to restrict the free access to the

Non-MR Personnel. Only zone I has free access to the general public. Zone II is made for patient history and preparation. Zone III should be physically restricted from general public access. Only MR personnel will have free access to zone III. Zone IV is the MR scanner room itself and located within the zone III. Non-MR personnel are not allowed to enter zones III and IV without prior screening.

MR Personnel/Non-MR Personnel

MR personnel are those who have been trained and educated about MR safety and approved by the MR Medical Director of the institution or the center. Only MR personnel should have free access to zones III and IV.

Screening of Patient and Non-MR Personnel

MR personnel should screen patients and relatives for any metallic, ferromagnetic objects before allowing entry into zone III and IV. They should be asked to remove metallic personal belongings and devices such as watches, jewellery, pagers, mobiles phones, body piercings, contraceptive diaphragms, metallic drug delivery patches, clothing items that may contain fasteners, hooks, zippers, loose metallic components or metallic threads, cosmetic containing metallic particles such as eye makeups. Metallic devices can be screened with hand-held magnet (>1000 gauss). Any person with suspected metallic foreign body in the orbit or near vital organs should be investigated with plain radiographs and if required CT scan. Intraocular foreign body is an absolute contraindication for undergoing MR examination. With metallic implants, materials and foreign body the possible adverse effect include displacement, induction of electric current in the object, excessive heating causing burns and misinterpretation because of artifacts.

Pregnancy-Related Issues

Electromagnetic fields used for MRI have the potential to produce developmental abnormalities. It can affect cell undergoing divisions, as in developing fetus. However, there is little data available at present on this issue.

Pregnant Health Care Practitioner

Pregnant MR personnel can be permitted to work in and around the MR environment throughout all stages of pregnancy. However, they should be requested not to remain inside scanner room during actual data acquisition (when sequence is running). This should be specifically avoided during first three months of pregnancy.

Pregnant Patient

ACR white paper permits scanning of pregnant patient in any stage of pregnancy. It also suggests case-by-case analysis to decide whether data obtained by MR examination will significantly affect the patient management and whether this data can be obtained by any other modality.

Since there is no enough data available on MR safety during pregnancy scanning pregnant patient during first three months of pregnancy should be avoided.

Contrast Media during Pregnancy

Gadolinium is known to cross the placenta. It is then excreted by fetal kidney and can re-circulate through amniotic fluid several times. Gadolinium can dissociate from its chelate. ACR white paper recommends that MR contrast medium should not be injected in pregnant patient. However, a case-by-case basis decision can be done of risk-benefit analysis.

Contrast Media in Lactating Patients

Gadolinium is excreted in human milk. Breast milk should be expressed after injection and thrown away. Baby should not be breast fed for 36-48 hours.

Aneurysm and Hemostatic Clips

Many of these clips in use are ferromagnetic and they are absolute contraindication for MR examination. Only those aneurysm clips that are tested prior to placement to be non-ferromagnetic and that are made up of titanium, and this is documented in writing by referring physician can undergo MR examination. Having safely undergone a prior MR examination with an aneurysm clip or other implant in place at any given static magnetic field strength is not in and of itself sufficient evidence of its MR safety or compatibility. Variation in static and gradient magnetic field can result into untoward effects next time.

Dental Devices and Materials

Lesser chances of displacement with these devices hence not an contraindication. However, artifacts caused by them can be problematic.

Heart Valves

Majority of prosthetic valves show measurable deflection forces. However, the deflection forces were relatively insignificant compared with the forces exerted by the beating heart. Therefore, patients with prosthetic heart valves may safely undergo MRI.

Intravascular Coils, Filters and Stents

These devices are usually attached firmly into the vessel wall approximately 4-6 weeks after deployment, therefore unlikely to be dislodged after 6 weeks. Patient may undergo MRI safely.

Ocular Implants

There is possibility of discomfort and minor injury with ocular implants. Risk-benefit analysis should be done.

Orthopedic Implants, Materials and Devices

Most of these devices used in present practice are made from non-ferromagnetic materials, therefore may be safely imaged by MRI. However, artifacts caused by them can be a problem, if they are in region of interest.

Otologic Implants

Cochlear implant is an absolute contraindication to undergo MR examination.

Pellets, Bullets and Sharpnels

Decision should be taken on individual basis with respect to position of the object near a vital neural, vascular or soft tissue structure. Assessment should be done by taking proper history and plain radiographs.

Penile Implants and Artificial Sphincters

Penile implants are relative contraindication for MR examination as they can cause patient discomfort. Artificial sphincters are absolute contraindication.

Pacemakers

Cardiac pacemakers are absolute contraindication for undergoing MR examination. There is possibility of displacement and damage of pacemaker, programming change, electromagnetic interference and fibrillation when patient with cardiac pacemaker undergoes MR examination.

Vascular Access Ports

Insignificant displacement of simple ports, hence not a contraindication. However, ports with electronic activation and programming are strict contraindication.

Patient Monitoring and Emergency

Monitoring devices like pulse oxymeter, ventilators are now available as MR compatible devices that can be used safely in scanner room. These should be kept as away from magnet bore as possible. In-spite of availability of these devices the first approach in case of emergency must be shifting the patient out of scanning room as early as possible and start resuscitation.

PRECAUTIONS

1. Always screen the patient and accompanying person for any metallic objects. Metallic objects can form projectile because of strong magnetic attraction. This can lead to life threatening consequences.
2. Always see to it that wires and coils are well insulated and are not touching patient's body. It can cause burns. Patient's body part should also not be touching magnet bore.
3. Avoid loop formation: Wires of pulse oxymeter, ECG leads etc should never form a loop. Loop formation can lead to induction of current and burns. Even loop formation of body parts for example crossed arms or legs can form a large conductive loop and can result into induction of current.
4. In case of emergency first approach must be to remove the patient out of scanner room as early as possible and start resuscitation.
5. Doors of scanner room should have label with pictures of object that are strictly prohibited to take inside scanner room.

ABSOLUTE CONTRAINDICATIONS

1. Internal cardiac pacemakers
2. Implantable cardiac defibrillators
3. Cochlear implants
4. Neurostimulators
5. Bone growth stimulators
6. Electrically programmed drug infusion pumps, vascular access ports
7. Intraocular foreign body
8. Aneurysm clips

CHAPTER 8

MR Contrast Media

INTRODUCTION

In the beginning years of MR imaging, it was thought that MR may not need any contrast medium injection because of its inherent tissue contrast. Soon it was found that contrast enhancement improves detection, delineation and characterisation, and increases confidence in the interpretation. Now with fast sequences like EPI available, it is possible to do physiological and dynamic studies like perfusion.

CLASSIFICATION OF MR CONTRAST MEDIA

1. Parenteral
2. Oral

Parenteral agents can be classified based on relaxivity and susceptibility.

Depending on Relaxivity

1. Positive relaxation agents (T1 agents)
   These agents affect T1 relaxation and reduce T1 of the tissue in which they accumulate. This results into increase in signal intensity on T1-W images hence these agents are called positive relaxation agents.
   Examples: Gadolinium, Mn-DPDP.
2. Negative relaxation agents (T2 agents)
   They affect T2 relaxation and reduce T2 of the tissue where they accumulate. The result is reduction in signal intensity of the tissue on T2-W images.
   Examples: Iron oxide particles, gadolinium.

Depending on Susceptibility

1. Paramagnetic agents
   Gadolinium is a paramagnetic agent. They are usually positive agents but at higher doses can cause T2 shortening resulting into decreased signal on T2-W images. When paramagnetic agents initially pass through vascular bed of brain, they cause local T2 shortening and decrease in signal on T2-W images. This effect is used in perfusion studies.
2. Superparamagnetic and ferromagnetic agents
   They are negative agents. They cause spin dephasing leading to T2 shortening and signal loss. Example: Iron oxide (Fe_3O_4).

Mechanism of MR Contrast Enhancement

In X-ray/CT contrast is related to only one factor- degree of X-ray attenuation caused by electron density of tissues or contrast agent. In MR the mechanism is multi-factorial and include spin density, relaxivity (T1, T2), magnetic susceptibility, diffusion and perfusion of contrast agent.

Relaxivity

Paramagnetic ions increase relaxation of water protons by dipole-dipole relaxation. The phenomenon by which excited protons are affected by nearby excited protons or electrons is called 'dipole-dipole interaction'. This dipole-dipole interaction affects rotational and translational diffusion of water molecules leading to their relaxation. The more and closer water molecules approach the paramagnetic ions, greater will be relaxation (Fig. 8.1).

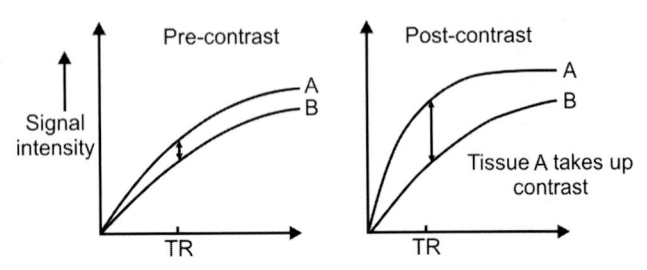

Fig. 8.1: T1 curves-pre- and post-contrast: Tissue A takes up gadolinium leading to reduction in its T1 and increased signal intensity. At short TR the signal intensity difference between A and B increases resulting into increased contrast

Gadolinium (Gd)

Gd is rare earth metal of lanthanide group with atomic number 64. Free Gd ions tend to accumulate in body and do not get excreted. This can result into toxicity. To prevent this toxicity Gd ions are combined with chelates that cause their rapid and total renal excretion.

Gd leads to both T1 and T2 relaxation. Increased T1 relaxation leads to bright signal on T1-W images. T1 effects of Gd are used more commonly for clinical purposes. T2 effects of Gd leading to reduction in T2 and decreased signal on T2-W and PD images, is clinically not relevant. However, susceptibility effects (not relaxivity) of Gd as it initially passes through vascular bed leads to decreased signal on T2-W images. This effect is used in MR perfusion.

MR CONTRAST MEDIA

Gadolinium

Atomic number-64

Paramagnetic agent

Reduces T1 and T2 of the tissues where it accumulates. Increased signal on T1-w and reduced signals on T2-w images.

Usual dose: 0.1 mmol/kg

Median lethal dose (LD50): 6-30 mmol/kg

Overall adverse reaction rate: 3-5%.

Osmolality:

Ionic: Magnevist – 1960 mmol/kg

Nonionic: Omniscan –   789 mmol/kg

              ProHance –   620 mmol/kg

Gadolinium Chelates

Chelates are substances that have high affinity for metal ions. They bind with metal ions and make them less toxic and facilitate their excretion.

Two groups of chelates:

I. Linear:
   1. Gd-DTPA—Gadopentetate dimeglumine (Magnevist, Magniscan)
   2. Gd-DTPA-BMA—Gadodiamide (Omniscan)
   3. Gd-DTPA-bismethoxyethylamide, Gadoversatamide (Optimark)

II. Macrocyclic (Ring):
   1. Gd-HP-DO3A—Gadoteridol (ProHance)
   2. Gd-DOTA—Gadoterate meglumine (Dotarem)
   3. Gd-DO3A-botrol—gadobutrol (Gadovist)

Hepatobiliary Chelates

They are taken up by hepatocytes and excreted in part in bile.
1. Gd-BOPTA (Gadobenate dimeglumine)
2. Gd-EOB-BOPTA

Adverse Reactions

Majority of adverse reactions to Gd are mild and transient. Overall reaction rate is 3-5% and include nausea, headache. Anaphylaxis is very rare. Patient with history of allergy, asthma, previous reaction to drugs, iodinated contrast, Gd are more prone for the adverse reactions. Precautions should be taken in these cases. Reversible increase in serum iron and bilirubin can be seen. Ionic versus non-ionic MR contrast is not as significant clinically as in iodinated contrast.

Safety Issues

1. Renal failure
   Safety is not clearly established in renal failure although it is well tolerated. Gd chelates can be dialysed.
2. History of allergy/asthma
   Precautions should be taken in these patients with constant monitoring. Pre-medications like hydrocortisone and antihistaminic drugs can be injected beforehand.
3. Pregnancy
   Gadolinium is known to cross the placenta. It is then excreted by fetal kidney and can re-circulate through

amniotic fluid several times. Gadolinium can dissociate from its chelate. ACR white paper recommends that MR contrast medium should not be injected in pregnant patient. However, a case-by-case basis decision can be done of risk-benefit analysis.

4. Lactation

    Gadolinium is excreted in human milk. Breast milk should be expressed after injection and thrown away. Baby should not be breast fed for 36-48 hours.

Other MR Contrast Agents

1. Iron Oxide (Fe_3O_4) is a superparamagnetic agent. It is phagocytosed by reticuloendothelial system (RES) with prominent uptake in liver and spleen. Focal areas such as metastases do not have RES so they remain same while normal liver tissue takes up Iron oxide and become dark on T2-W image. Hence metastases appear relatively bright.

2. Mn-DPDP (Magnafodipir trisodium)

    It causes positive contrast enhancement on T1-W images in liver.

3. Dysprosium Chelates: Dy-HP-DO3A

    These were found to be more superior to Gd chelates in perfusion studies (not in routine T1-W images) because of more T2 relaxivity and susceptibility effects.

Oral Contrast Agents

1. Positive contrast

    Example: Manganese chloride, Gd-DTPA, oil emulsions
    Image degradation can occur with peristaltic movements of bowel.

122 MRI MADE EASY (FOR BEGINNERS)

2. Negative contrast
   They decrease signal from bowel lumen, therefore, there is no motion related image degradation.
   Example: Superparamagnetic iron oxide particle reduce signal by susceptibility effects. Barium, Blue-berry juice, PFOB are also used to reduce signals from bowel.

ROLE OF CONTRAST IN MRI

It has been shown that there is substantial improvement in lesion identification and characterisation with Gd.

CNS Neoplasm: Contrast improves identification, margin delineation and invasion in brain tumors (Figs 8.2A and B). It is must in patients undergoing surgery. Metastases and meningiomas can appear isointense on plain scan. Contrast

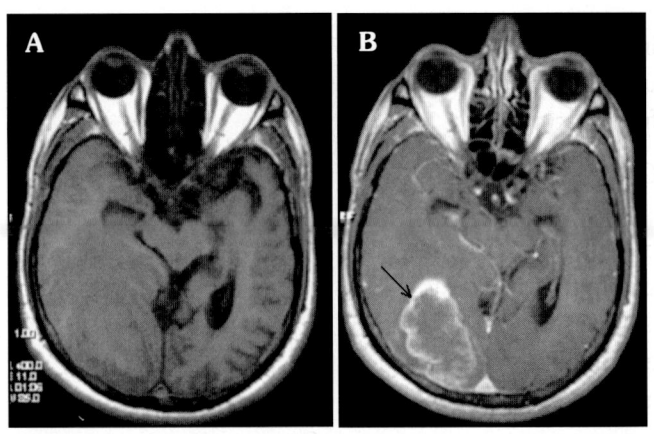

Figs 8.2A and B: Brain tumor: A. Precontrast T1-w axial image of the brain shows a large ill-defined space occupative lesion in right occipital region. B. Post-contrast image shows predominantly peripheral enhancement (arrows)

MR CONTRAST MEDIA 123

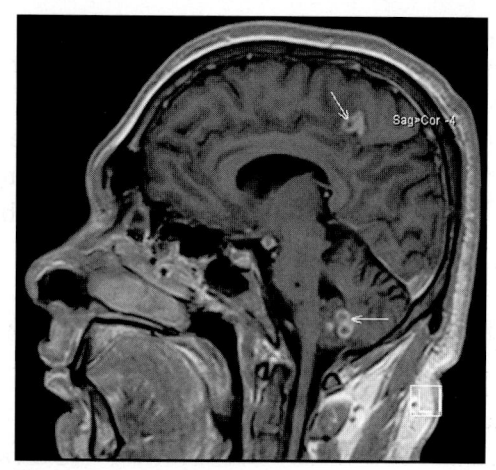

Fig. 8.3: T1-w post-contrast sagittal image of the brain shows multiple ring enhancing lesions (arrows) suggestive of tuberculomas

injection makes them more conspicuous. Contrast is very useful in post treatment tumors to differentiate recurrence from necrosis, specially with MR perfusion.

CNS Infection: Contrast enables lesion characterisation and assessment of lesion activity (Fig. 8.3). Acute lesions may be differentiated from chronic lesions (gliosis). Disease progression/regression can be monitored. Enhanced MRI is superior to enhanced CT specially in meningeal enhancement (Fig. 8.4) because of beam hardening artifacts in CT.

Ischemic CNS diseases: Gd is not routinely indicated in ischemic diseases. However, it can be useful for temporal dating and characterisation. Intravascular enhancement is

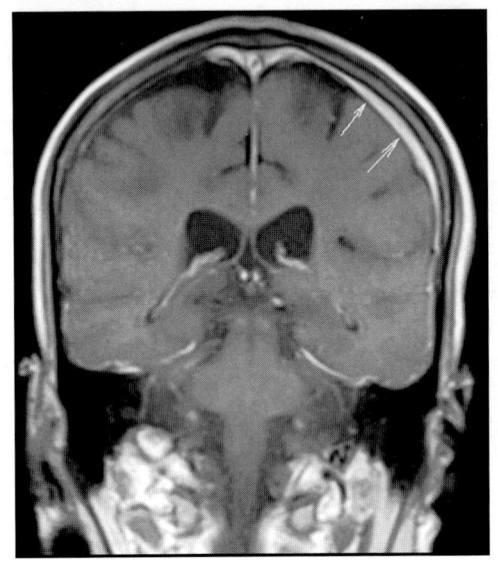

Fig. 8.4: T1-w post-contrast coronal image of the brain shows thick asymmetric enhancement of the meninges along the left parietal convexity (arrows)

seen in first week after infarction, with parenchymal enhancement seen after that upto 8 weeks. Intravascular and gyriform enhancement may help differentiating infarct from other conditions.

Spine: Contrast injection is indicated in postoperative spine to differentiate between scar and disc. Scar being a vascular structure enhances while disc usually does not enhance as it is a non-vascular structure (Figs 8.5A and B). Gd increases visualisation of leptomeningeal metastases and may differentiate tumor syrinx from congenital/traumatic syrinx. In vertebral body metastases Gd injection can be avoided as it does not improve the lesion characterisation.

MR CONTRAST MEDIA 125

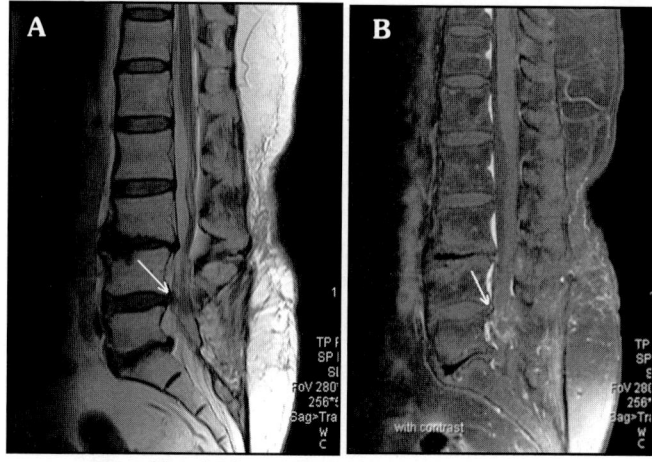

Figs 8.5A and B: Postoperative spine
A. T2-W sagittal image of the spine shows prominent disc herniation at L4-5 level. Note evidence of laminectomy at the same level.
B. T1-W post contrast sagittal image of the spine shows that the disc at L4-5 is not enhancing (arrow)

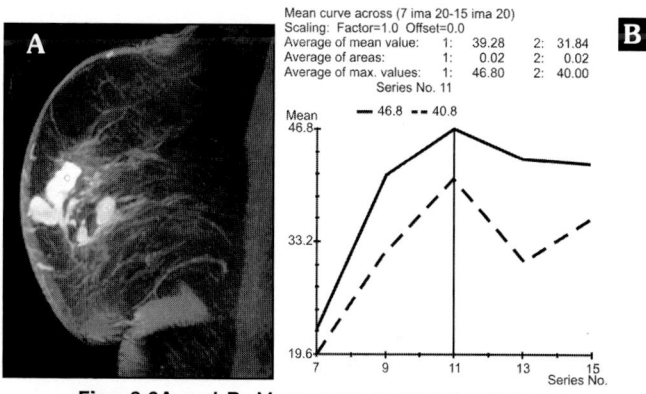

Figs 8.6A and B: Mean curve in breast malignancy
A. T1-W post-contrast sagittal image of the breast shows enhancing nodules
B. Mean curve analysis shows that there is rapid uptake-rapid washout of contrast suggestive of probably malignant lesion

Body Imaging: Eventhough body MR imaging has high intrinsic tissue contrast, Gd is useful in viable versus necrotic lesion, for identification of active infection and in recurrent neoplasm. It may help in differentiating benign from malignant lesions. Gd is used in breast (Figs 8.6A and B), liver, spleen, kidney and musculoskeletal pathologies, specially neoplastic. Gd is used in stress perfusion and myocardial viability in cardiac MRI.

CHAPTER 9

Principles of Interpretation: Neuroimaging

To be able to interpret MR images, apart from detail anatomical and pathological knowledge, knowing basics of pulse sequence and their specific uses is essential.

SIGNAL INTENSITY

Signal intensity of any structure depends on density of protons (hydrogen ions) in that structure, longitudinal relaxation time (T1), transverse relaxation time (T2) and flow and diffusion effects. Most intense signals are received from tissues with short T1 and long T2 and high proton concentration. Conversely, lowest signal intensity is seen in tissues with long T1, short T2 and low proton concentration. All these factors decide appearance of the structure/lesion on particular sequence. Water has long T1 and long T2 and appears dark on T1-weighted and bright on T2-weighted images. Fat has short T1 and short T2 and appears bright on T1-weighted and less bright on T2-weighted images. Inspite of its short T2, fat does not turn dark on T2-weighted images because of its high proton content.

Air is always dark/black on all sequences because of very low hydrogen proton concentration. Cortical bone is also dark on both T1 and T2-weighted images because of very low mobile protons. Appearance of medullary bone depends on the degree of fat replacement. Circulating blood in the vessels will be seen as flow void (dark) in all spin echo sequences and bright on gradient echo sequences. (for the mechanism refer to chapter on MR Angiography).

Calcifications are usually dark on both T1 and T2-weighted images with some exceptions. Lesions having high content of protenaceous material, methemoglobin (subacute hemorrhage) and cholesterol debries appear bright on T1-weighted images. Some lesions of basal ganglion that are bright on T1-weighted images include hyperintense globi palladi in hepatocellular degeneration, manganese deposition in parenteral nutrion, some cacifications and neurofibromatosis.

Normally, white matter (WM) is bright on T1-weighted images as compared to gray matter (GM) because of myelin (lipid) content of WM. On T2-weighted images GM, because of its more water content, has high signal intensity than WM. Posterior pituitary is seen as bright signal on T1-weighted images because of neurosecretary granules (Fig. 9.1). Presence of the bright posterior pituitary on T1-weighted images is related to the functional status of the hypothalamoneurohypophyseal axis. In adult patients clivus should be seen as homogeneous high signal intensity on T1-w images because of its fatty marrow content.

SEQUENCE SELECTION

Whatever the reason for scanning few basic sequences are run in all brain examinations. They include T2-w axial, Diffusion, T1-w sagittal, gradient Hemo, Flair- axial, and T2-w coronal. Conventionally, T1-weighted images are used to see anatomy and T2-weighted images show pathologies well. Majority of pathologies are associated with increased T1 and T2 relaxation times with edema

130 MRI MADE EASY (FOR BEGINNERS)

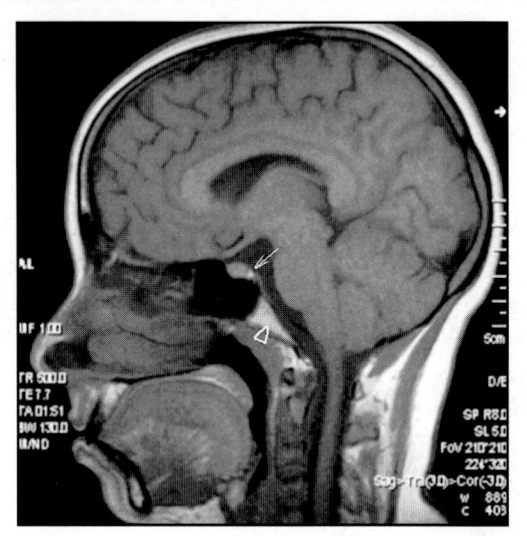

Fig. 9.1: T1-w sagittal image of the brain. Posterior pituitary is seen as bright signal in the sella (arrow). Note the bright homogenous clivus (arrowhead) as it contains fatty marrow. Also appreciate the white matter has higher signal intensity than gray matter

hence appear bright on T2-w images. Examination usually starts with T2-w images and can be tailored depending on what is seen on it.

STROKE IMAGING

Examination should start with diffusion images that will show acute infarct. Gradient- hemo sequence shows acute bleed and fast flair that shows subarachnoid haemorrhage, should be done next. Time of flight MR angiography can be done for the status of the vessels. If infarcts are peripheral

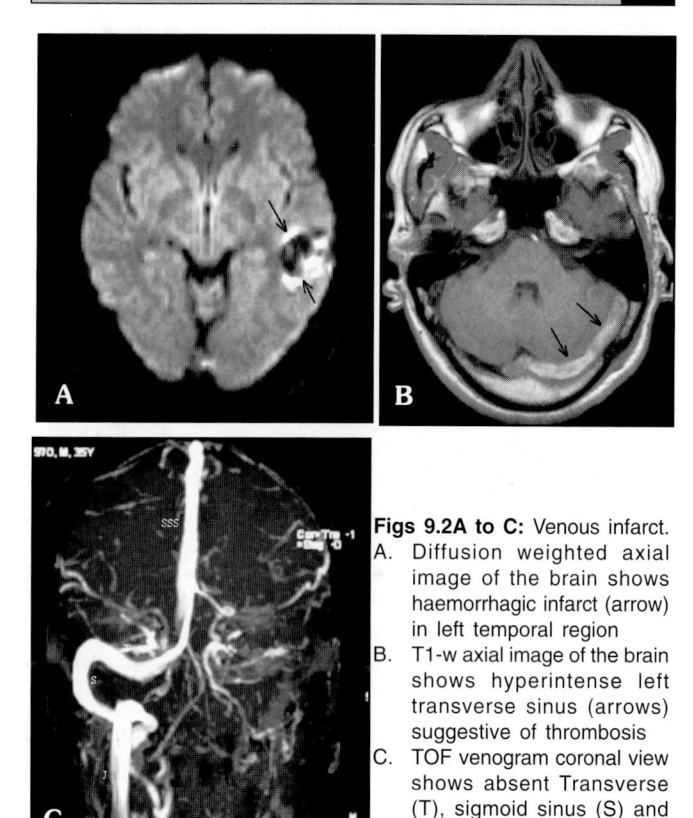

PRINCIPLES OF INTERPRETATION: NEUROIMAGING 131

Figs 9.2A to C: Venous infarct.
A. Diffusion weighted axial image of the brain shows haemorrhagic infarct (arrow) in left temporal region
B. T1-w axial image of the brain shows hyperintense left transverse sinus (arrows) suggestive of thrombosis
C. TOF venogram coronal view shows absent Transverse (T), sigmoid sinus (S) and Jugular vein (J)

and hemorrhagic, then phase contrast MR venograms are useful to rule out venous sinus thrombosis (Figs 9.2A to C). In case of posterior circulation stroke T1-w fat saturated axial sections of the neck are done to see for vertebral pathologies like dissection or thrombosis (Figs 9.3A to C).

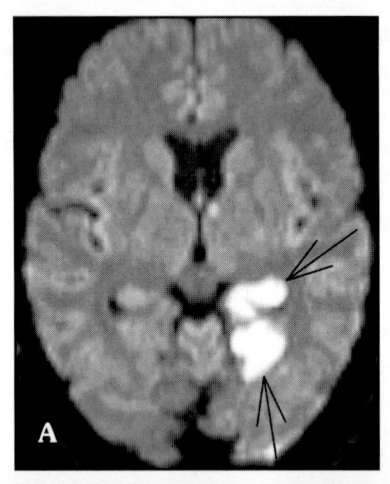

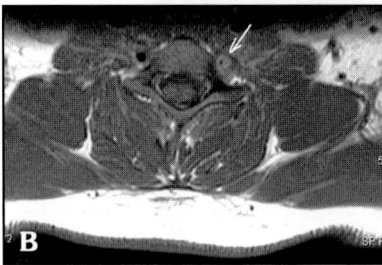

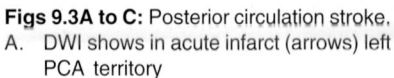

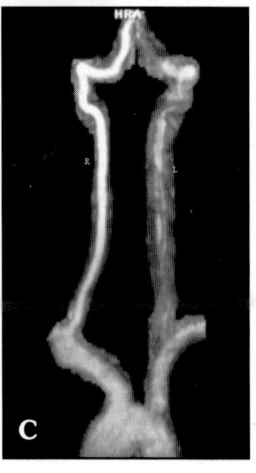

Figs 9.3A to C: Posterior circulation stroke.
A. DWI shows in acute infarct (arrows) left PCA territory
B. T1-w axial image of the neck shows vertebral artery dissection on left side (arrow)
C. Four vessel MR Angiogram shows dissected left vertebral artery (L)

Tumors

MR is the best modality to evaluate brain tumors because of its excellent soft tissue contrast and multiplanar capability.

Intravenous gadolinium injection is must for evaluation of brain tumors. Tumor enhancement suggest break in the blood-brain barrier and do not represent tumor vascularity (Figs 9.4A to D). Tumor vascularity is evaluated with MR perfusion. MR perfusion and spectroscopy can be helpful in 1. differentiating neoplastic from non-neoplastic lesions, 2. grading of tumors and 3. guidance for the biopsy. Spinal cord screening should be done in tumors like ependymoma, medulloblastoma, hemangioblastoma, choroids plexus tumors to rule out 'drop metastases'.

Infection

As in tumor intravenous gadolinium injection is must in evaluation of CNS infection. Contrast enhanced MR is superior to contrast enhanced CT because it shows dural enhancement and thickening better (Fig. 9.5). However, MR is inferior to CT in chronic and congenital infectious processes with calcifications as major finding.

Epilepsy

Apart from routine imaging to rule out SOL, the area of focus in epilepsy specially partial complex seizure (associated with loss of consciousness) is temporal lobe and hippocampus. The imaging of hippocampus should involve oblique coronal sections that are roughly parallel to the anterior surface of the pons such that hippocampus is seen in true cross section. Side-to-side symmetry of the hippocampus for comparison is judged by cochlea appearing symmetrical on a single image. Oblique coronal

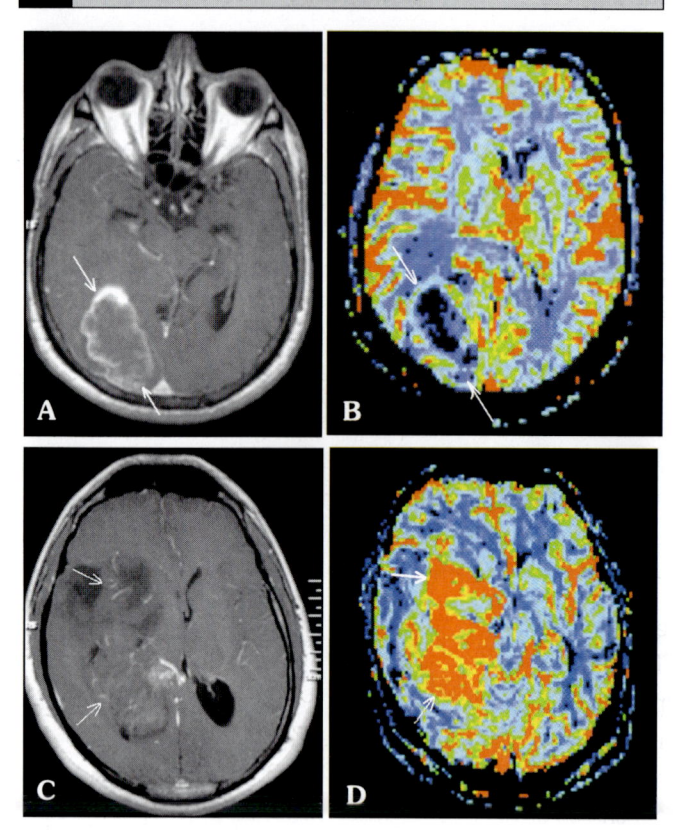

Figs 9.4A to D: Tumor vascularity

A. T1-w post contrast axial image of the brain shows enhancing tumor in the right occipital lobe (arrows)
B. Perfusion image CCBV map shows the lesion to be hypovascular (arrows). Red area correspond with high perfusion while blue or dark is suggestive of least perfusion
C. T1-w post-contrast axial image of the brain shows predominantly non-enhancing tumor in the right cerebral hemisphere (arrows) causing mass effect and midline shift
D. Perfusion image CCBV map shows the lesion to be hypervascular (arrows)

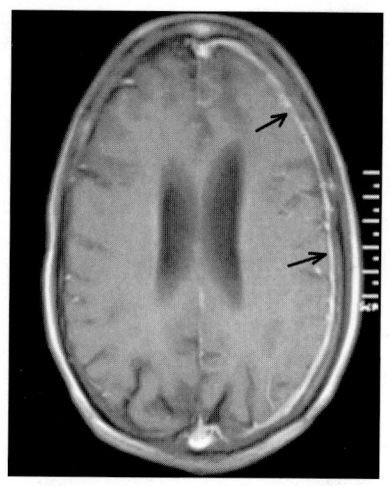

Fig. 9.5: T1-w post-contrast axial image of the brain shows enhancing meninges along left cerebral hemisphere (arrows)

sequences (Figs 9.6A to C) include T2-w, FLAIR, medium TI inversion recovery and flash T1 3D. FLAIR shows small epileptogenic foci in the cortex and signal abnormalities in mesial temporal sclerosis. Medium TI inversion recovery shows cortical dysplasia and migrational abnormalities well as it shows gray-white differentiation best. It is also good for hippocampal architecture. T2-weighted gradient hemo sequence should be included to see any subtle haemorrhages associated with small vascular malformations and trauma. MR findings of mesial temporal sclerosis alone or in combination are hippocampal atrophy, increased signals on T-2 or FLAIR images and loss of internal architecture.

136 MRI MADE EASY (FOR BEGINNERS)

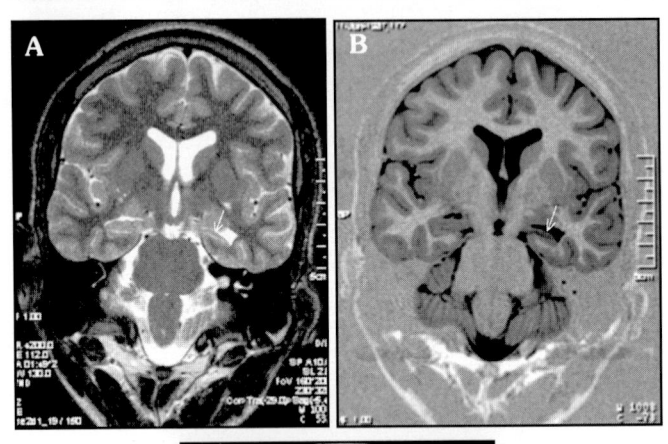

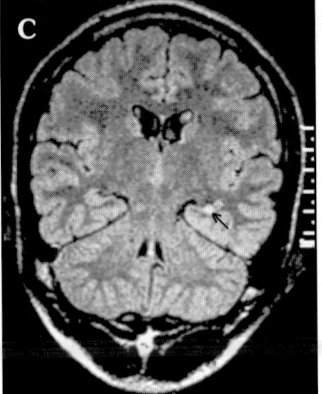

Figs 9.6A to C: Epilepsy protocol
A. T2-w oblique coronal image of the temporal lobes shows the left hippocampus to be atrophic (arrow). Note increased size of temporal horn on the side
B. Medium TI IR sequence oblique coronal image of the temporal lobes shows the atrophic left hippocampus (arrow). Note gray white differentiation in this image
C. FLAIR oblique coronal image of the temporal lobes shows the atrophic as well as hyperintense left hippocampus (arrow)

These findings are suggestive left mesial temporal sclerosis

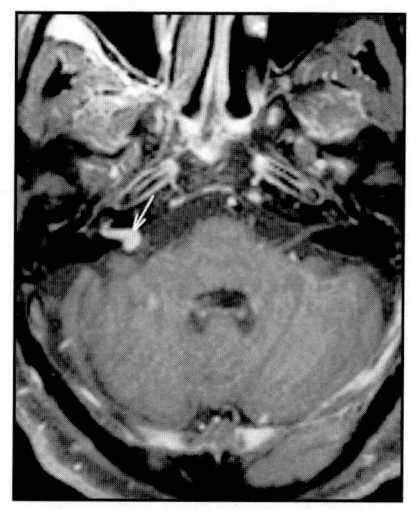

PRINCIPLES OF INTERPRETATION: NEUROIMAGING | **137**

Fig. 9.7: T1-w post contrast axial image of the brain shows small enhancing acoustic neuroma in the right internal auditory canal (arrow)

CP Angle Lesions

All patients presenting with tinnitus, hearing loss and vertigo should have a highly T2-w sequence called CISS that shows dark cranial nerves in bright CSF. Study should also include MR angiogram to rule out any vascular loop as a cause of tinnitus. Intravenous gadolinium is injected to rule out labrynthitis and any small enhancing acoustic neuroma in IAC (Fig. 9.7).

Demyelinating Lesions

T2-w images are mainstay for demyelinating lesions and should be acquired in all orthogonal planes. FLAIR images

138 MRI MADE EASY (FOR BEGINNERS)

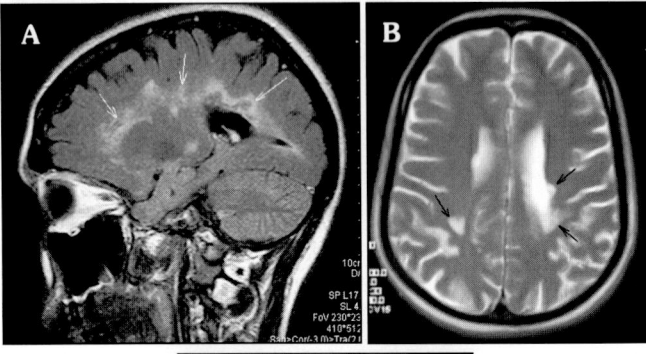

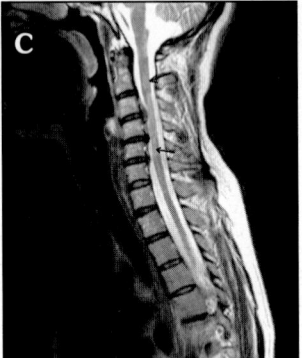

Figs 9.8A to C: Multiple sclerosis
A. FLAIR sagittal image of the brain shows multiple hyperintense plaques running vertically from corpus callosal margin (arrows) suggestive of 'Dowson's fingers'.
B. T2-w axial image of the brain shows multiple hyperintese plaques (arrows) in periventricular white matter.
C. T2-w sagittal image of the cervical spine shows hyperintense plaques in the cord (arrow).

show lesion near ventricular margin better by suppressing CSF. FLAIR sagittal images best show callaso-septal lesions and 'Dowson's finger' running perpendicular to the ventricular margin in multiple sclerosis (Figs 9.8A to C).

PRINCIPLES OF INTERPRETATION: NEUROIMAGING

Spinal cord should be screened in demyelinating lesions to rule cord involvement. Contrast is given in multiple sclerosis to see the activity of the lesion. Enhancing lesions are usually active.

Trauma

CT is still preferred over MRI for head injury. CT is convenient, less time consuming and available everywhere. It shows acute bleed and bony fractures easily. Gradient hemo and T1-weighted images are important in showing acute bleed. MR is useful in evaluation of diffuse axonal injury and sequelae of head injury (Fig. 9.9). MR is also useful when CT in indeterminate in posterior fossa lesions.

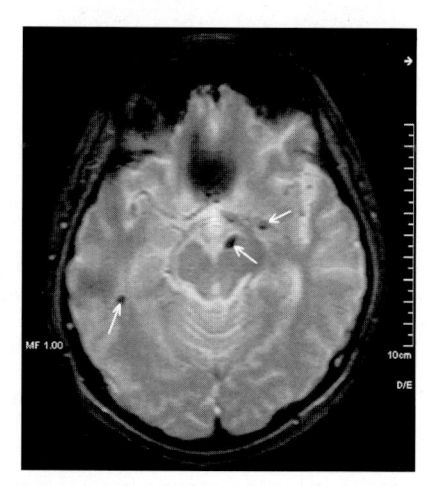

Fig. 9.9: Gradient Hemo axial image of the brain shows small petechial hemorrhages (arrows) in this head injury patient suggestive of diffuse axonal injury (DAI)

MRI in Pediatric Brain

Knowledge of stages of normal myelination is important. Myelination progresses caudocranially, dorsoventrally and center to periphery. It is usually completed by two years of age. Myelinated white matter appears bright on T1-w and dark on T2-w images (Figs 9.10A and B). The sequence that shows the suspected pathology best should be run first. MR is the modality of choice in pediatric brain tumors, congenital anomalies and hyoxic-ischemic injury (HIE) (Figs 9.11A and B). Correlation with perinatal and birth history is required as hypoxic-ischemic injury affects

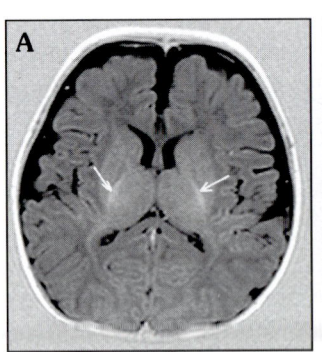

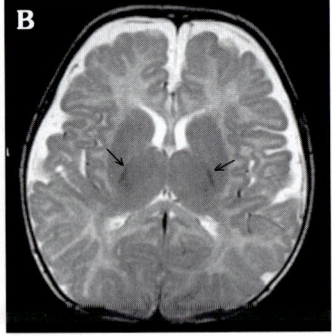

Figs 9.10A and B: Normal myelination in two months old infant
A. T1-w medium TI IR axial image of the brain shows myelination in the posterior limb of the internal capsule as bright linear structures (arrows).
B. T2-w axial image of the brain shows myelination in posterior limbs as dark structures (arrows)

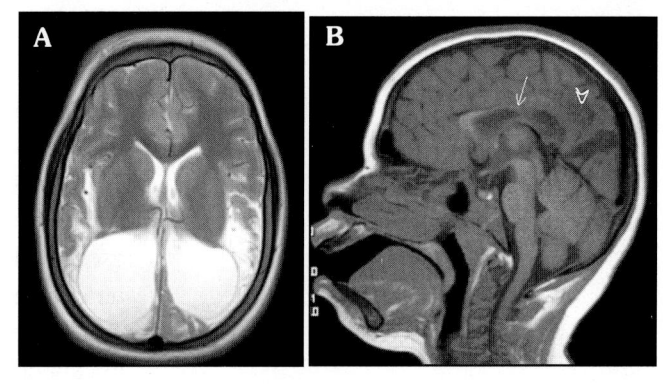

Figs 9.11A and B: Perinatal HIE/Hypoglycemic insult
A. T2-w axial image of the brain shows severe volume loss in occipito-parietal lobes with exvacio dilatation of the lateral ventricles.
B. T1-w sagittal image of the brain shows severe volume loss (arrowhead) in the occipital region with severe atrophy of posterior part of corpus callosum (arrow).
This is a classical feature of perinatal hypoglycemic/hypoxic-ischemic insult.

periventricular white matter in premature infants while gray matter and water-shed areas are affected in term infants. Diffusion weighted images are useful in showing acute HIE. Metabolic diseases can be evaluated with MR spectroscopy.

CHAPTER 10

Principles of Interpretation: Body Imaging

INTRODUCTION

It took more time for MR to establish its role in body imaging as compared to neuroimaging. The main reason for this lag was movement artifacts caused by respiration (Fig. 10.1), cardiac pulsation and peristalsis. Now with improved pulse sequence design and gradient technology leading to ultrafast sequences like EPI, has made possible to image any organ or area with MRI. As far as musculoskeletal pathologies are concerned, MR is the modality of choice.

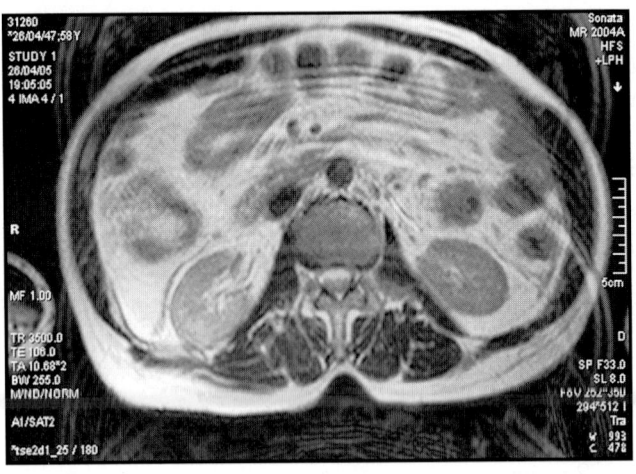

Fig. 10.1: T2-w axial image of the abdomen. Breathing artifacts are seen as multiple horizontal lines. Note the phase encoding direction from anterior to posterior

In this chapter few basic concepts behind musculoskeletal and body imaging are discussed.

SEQUENCES

Apart from T1-w and T2-w images, one sequence that has made impact on body and musculoskeletal imaging is STIR. It is short TI inversion recovery sequence in which fat gets suppressed. As majority of pathologies have increased water content, they stand out (bright) on STIR sequence. It can be used almost anywhere in the body. Fast sequences like HASTE, RARE and TrueFISP can acquire images within single breath-hold and are mainstay for chest, abdomen and cardiac imaging. Fat saturation techniques, artifact reduction techniques like respiratory gating, cardiac gating have almost eliminated movement artifacts.

Spine Imaging

It is the most frequently done MRI scan in any MR center. Vertebrae in adult patient are bright on T1-w images because of fatty marrow and moderate to hypointense on T2-w images. Annulus fibrosus is dark on all sequences because of low mobile proton density and acellular nature of fibrous tissue (Fig. 10.2). Nucleus pulposus because of its high water content is dark on T1-w images and bright on T2-w images. A central dark horizontal internuclear cleft in nucleus pulposus on T2-w images in normal in patients above 30 years of age. Ligaments are dark on all sequence. Spinal cord has higher signal than CSF on T1-w images and lower signal than CSF on T2-w images. Apart from T1-w (Fig. 10.3) and T2-w axial and sagittal images, STIR should be done in vertebral focal lesion,

146 MRI MADE EASY (FOR BEGINNERS)

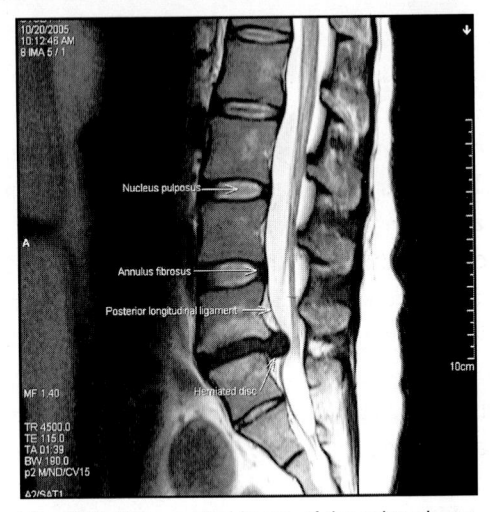

Fig. 10.2: T2-w sagittal image of the spine shows herniated disc at L4-5 level. Note other structures as labeled

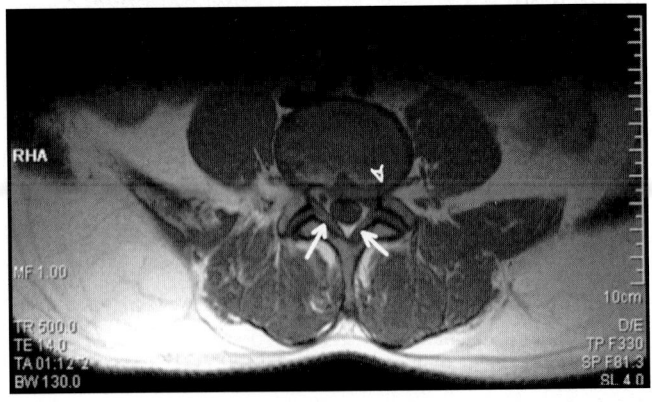

Fig. 10.3: T1-w axial image of the spine shows left posterolateral herniation of the disc encroaching on the neural foramina (arrowhead). Also see hypertrophy of ligamentum flavum (arrows)

trauma or marrow lesions. It is good idea to screen whole spine for the purpose of counting vertebrae. In a patient with low backache if L-S spine is normal then SI joint screening should be done as cause for the pain might be there. HASTE myelogram in lumbar spine gives gross idea of thecal sac in few seconds.

In post operative spine intravenous Gadolinium injection is must as it differentiate scar from recurrent disc prolapse. Scar being a vascular structure enhances in early phase while disc does not enhance in early phase (within 20-25 minutes). Some times scar and disc are mixed and disc can enhance because of infiltration by granulation tissue.

Marrow Imaging

MR is the most sensitive method for marrow imaging. Yellow marrow because of its fat content, is bright on T1-w images and moderate to iso-intense on T2-w images. Red marrow, which contains hematopoietic tissue, is iso to hypointense on T1 and T2-w images (Fig. 10.4). As child grows there is gradual conversion of red marrow into yellow marrow in appendicular to axial direction such that in adults red marrow is present only in axial skeleton like vertebrae, rib cage, sternum, skull and pelvis, and proximal metaphyses of femur and humerus. Epiphyses and apophyses almost never have red marrow and are last to reconvert into red marrow in hematopoietic crisis. So dark epiphyses and apophyses on T1-w images suggest severe hematopoietic disease. T1-w images are most useful in marrow evaluation. Red marrow has lower signal intensity

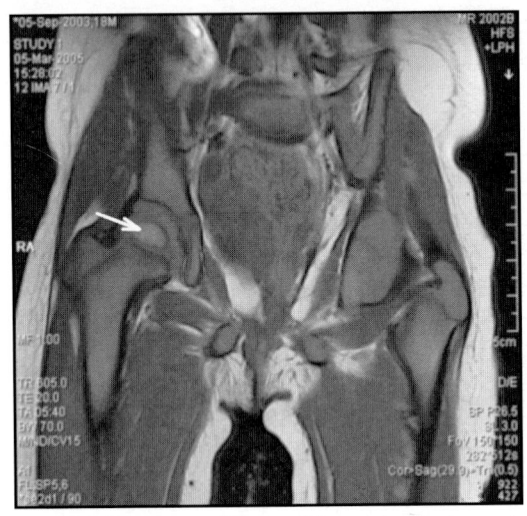

Fig. 10.4: T1-w coronal image of the pelvis. The femoral epiphysis is bright (arrow) as it contains fatty marrow

than fat but higher signal intensity than muscles. Marrow darker than that of muscle or intervertebral discs is always abnormal. Malignant lesions are either iso or dark than red marrow. STIR and other fat suppressed T1-w images are useful for marrow pathology. Marrow edema is best seen on STIR images (Fig. 10.5). Marrow involvement by neoplasm, infection or subtle trauma is earliest picked up by MRI specially with STIR sequence (Fig. 10.6). It requires more than 30% bone destruction to be visible on plain radiograph. Metastasis is seen as hypodense lesion in bright fatty marrow on T1-w images. This is not, however, specific appearance as myeloma, lymphoma or infective lesions are also dark on T1-w images.

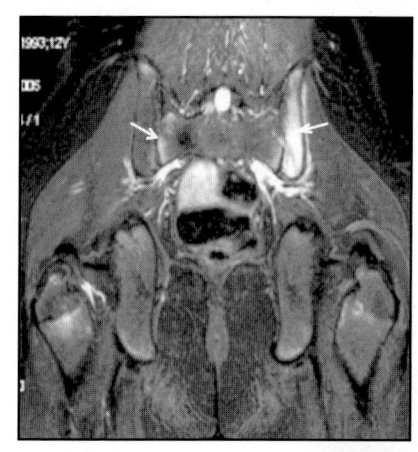

PRINCIPLES OF INTERPRETATION: BODY IMAGING 149

Fig. 10.5: STIR coronal image of the SI joints in patient of sacroiliatitis. Arrows indicate marrow edema

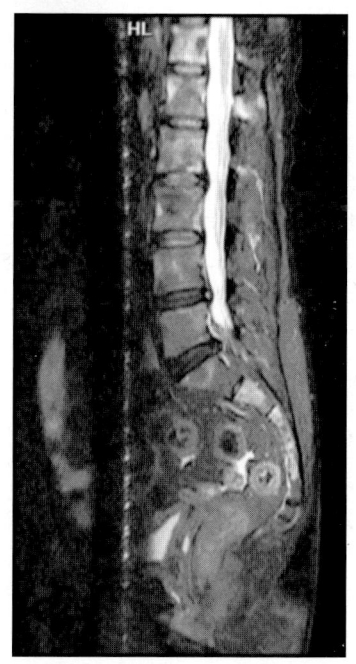

Fig. 10.6: STIR sagittal image of the lumbar spine shows multiple bright spots in vertebral bodies and posterior elements suggestive metastases

Musculoskeletal Neoplasms

MR plays important role in evaluating extent, staging and treatment planning in MS tumors. Cortical bone, ligament, tendon and fibrous tissue display low signal intensity on all sequences because of lack of mobile protons and relatively acellular matrix. Muscles have moderate signal intensity on T1-w and low signal intensity on T2-w images. Fat is bright on T1-w images and moderate signal intensity on T2-w images. Osteoid matrix is dark on all sequences while chondroid matrix shows moderate signal intensity on T1-w and high signal intensity on T2-w images (Figs 10.7A and B). Nonosseous tumors are usually low signal intensity on T1-w and high signal intensity on T2-w. These signal intensity characteristics are used to differentiate tumors and evaluating the extent and staging. Marrow involvement evaluated on T1-w and STIR images. The bone affected by the tumor should be screened in its entire extent by STIR sequence to rule out skip lesions. Intravenous contrast injection is must in musculoskeletal tumors as it improves depiction of lesion margin, presence of necrosis, cyst formation or drainable fluid collection and tumor vascularity assessment.

Joint Imaging

MR is mainstay for evaluation of joint pathologies as it shows ligaments, cartilages, joint effusion very well. Infection, neoplasm, trauma, arthritis are best evaluated with MR. Apart from T1 and T2-w images in orthogonal planes, PD, STIR and DESS sequences are used for joint

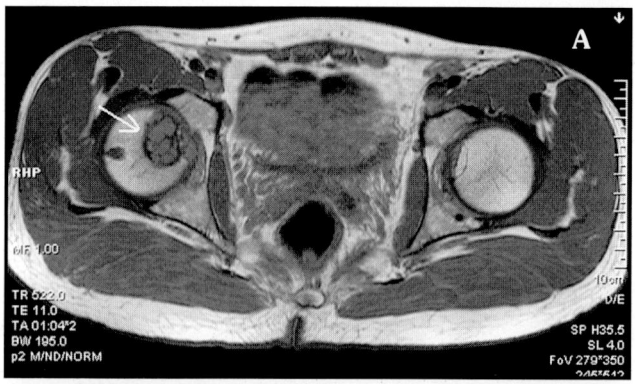

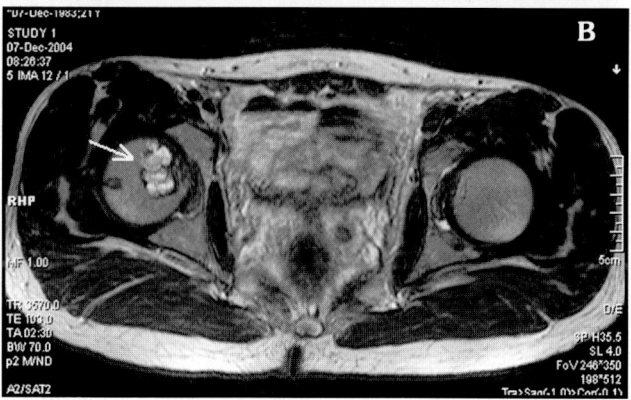

PRINCIPLES OF INTERPRETATION: BODY IMAGING | **151**

Figs 10.7A and B: Chondroid matrix
A. T1-w axial image of the pelvis shows dark lesion in the head of the right femur (arrow).
B. T2-w axial image of the pelvis shows the same lesion as bright lesion (arrow) because of its chondroid matrix.

imaging. STIR images show marrow edema, fluid collections, bursal inflammation. DESS is a steady state gradient echo sequence that shows articular cartilage as moderate signal intensity (Fig. 10.8). MR arthrogram can

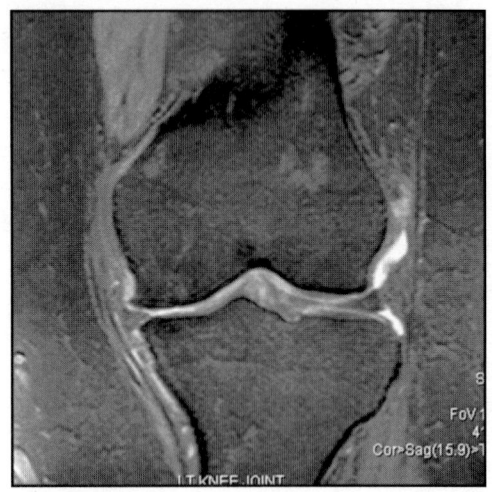

Fig. 10.8: DESS coronal image of the knee joint shows cartilage loss in the medial compartment. Compare with the lateral compartment. Osteophytes are also seen

be performed for recurrent dislocation of shoulder and Perthes disease of the hip joint for detailed evaluation of ligaments, joint capsule and articular cartilages.

Abdominal Imaging

Liver has shorter T1 and T2 relaxation times than spleen hence it is brighter than spleen on T1-w images and lower signal intensity than spleen on T2-w images. Iron or copper accumulation in liver makes it dark specially on T2 and T2*-w images.

MRCP has become an important non-invasive method to evaluate biliary and pancreatic tree. Heavily T2-w fast

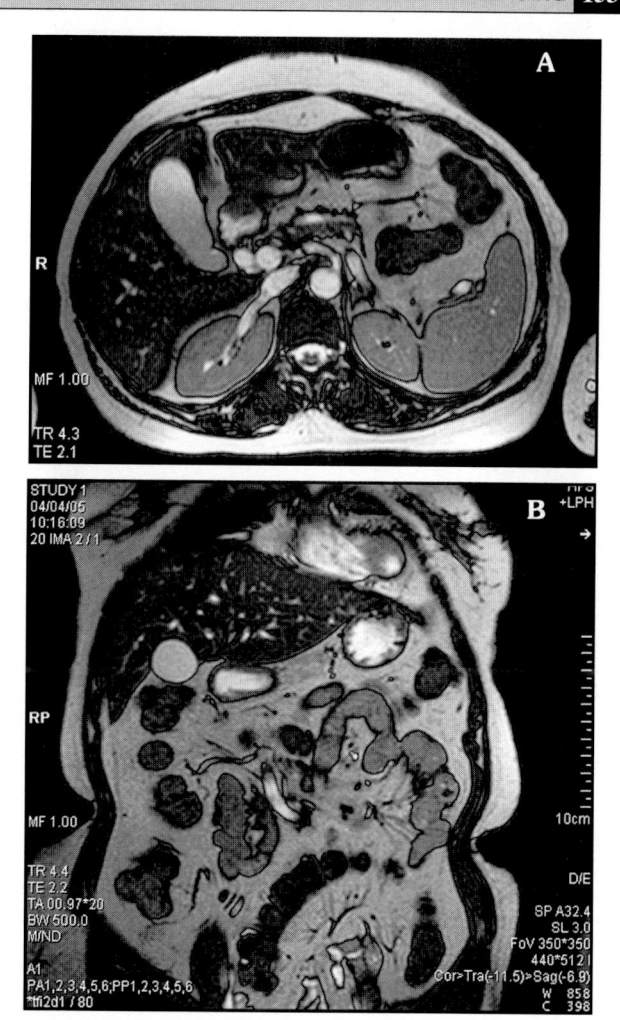

PRINCIPLES OF INTERPRETATION: BODY IMAGING 153

Figs 10.9A and B: MR abdominal imaging. True FISP axial (A) and coronal (B) images in a normal patient

sequences like HASTE and RARE are used for MRCP. These sequences are also used to evaluate other slow moving or stable fluids like ureters in MR urogram and thecal sac in MR myelogram. Gradient echo steady state sequence True FISP acquires good quality images of abdomen (Figs 10.9A and B) and chest in single breath-hold. T1- w FLASH images can be used for pre- and post-contrast imaging of abdomen. Triple-phase study of liver lesion can be performed with these sequences in patient where CT is contraindicated.

Pelvic Imaging

MR has surpassed CT in evaluation of pelvic pathologies, both in male and female pelvis. It is the best modality to stage tumors of urinary bladder, prostate and uterus. Prostate zonal anatomy is well seen on T2-w images. Inner transitional/central zone is seen as lower signal intensity than peripheral zone that is bright (Fig. 10.10). Any low signal intensity focus in peripheral bright zone in an old patient usually represents carcinoma prostate.

T2-w images again are useful in depicting anatomy of urinary bladder wall. Bladder wall is seen as low signal intensity smooth structure as against high signal intensity of urine (Figs 10.11A and B). Visualisation of the low signal intensity line between tumor and perivesical fat is an important feature in MR staging, differentiating T3a from T3b stage. Papillary intraluminal growth, however, are well seen as high signal intensity lesions in dark urine on T1-w images.

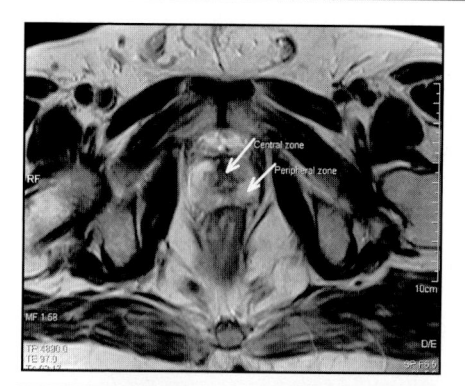

PRINCIPLES OF INTERPRETATION: BODY IMAGING 155

Fig. 10.10: Prostate imaging. T2-w axial image of the prostate shows dark central zone and bright peripheral zone

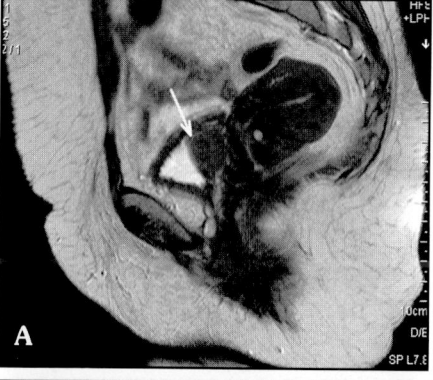

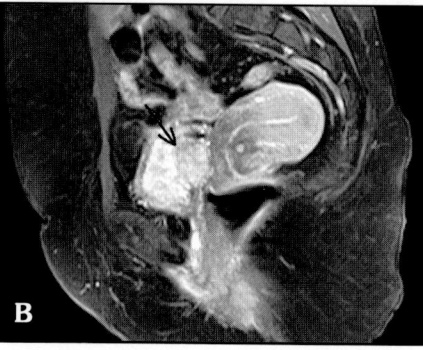

Figs 10.11A and B: Bladder imaging.
A. T2-w sagittal image of the pelvis shows a well-defined mass along the posterior wall of the urinary bladder (arrow).
B. Post-contrast T1-w sagittal image shows the enhancement in the mass (arrow). This mass turned out to be leiomyoma

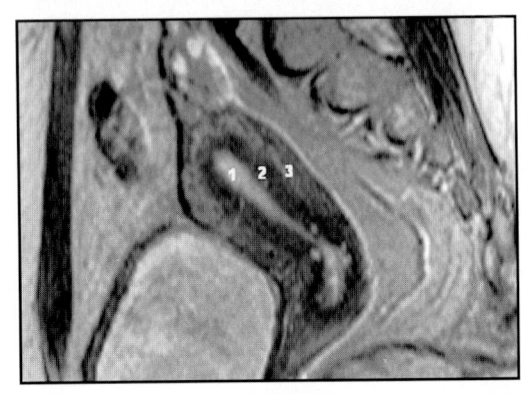

Fig. 10.12: Uterine imaging. Trilaminar pattern. 1-Endometrium, 2-Junctional zone-inner myometrium, and 3-Outer myometrium

Characteristic trilaminar zonal architecture of adult uterus seen on T2-w (Fig. 10.12) has helped to stage uterine carcinomas better. The normal endometrium and endometrial cavity are seen as high signal intensity central endometrial stripe. Intermediate low signal intensity junctional zone represents an inner layer of myometrium containing increased number of myometrial cells and increased density of compact muscle fibres. Peripheral zone is of intermediate signal intensity and represents outer myometrium. The same pattern continues into the cervix. However, an extra-layer of low signal intensity may be seen surrounding bright endometrial stripe on high resolution images probably representing mucosa and infolded plica palmatae.

Section II

CHAPTER 11

MR Angiography

INTRODUCTION

Lack of contrast injection, radiation and invasiveness makes MR angiography an attractive option for vascular assessment. Role of MR in vascular imaging is increasing day-by-day with technological advancement. The most recent application of MR reported is MR cineagiography analogous to X-ray catheter angiography.

MR angiography is based on flow information rather than morphological imaging in conventional angiography. So, it gives anatomical as well as hemodynamic information.

BLACK BLOOD IMAGING

In this blood appears black and sequence used is spin-echo sequence (Fig. 11.1). In spin-echo sequence nuclei that receive both 90° and 180° pulses will produce signal. However, flowing blood usually do not receive either 90 or 180 degree pulse. Hence, signal is not produced and flowing blood appears dark. Slow flow, clot, occlusion will show signal because it will receive both 90 degree excitation pulse and 180 degree rephasing pulse.

BRIGHT BLOOD IMAGING

In this type of imaging blood appears bright. Blood can be made bright by gradient echo sequence (Fig. 11.2) and intravascular contrast media.

In gradient echo sequence excitation pulse is slice selective. But rephasing, which is done by gradients rather than 180 degree pulse as in spin-echo sequence, is applied

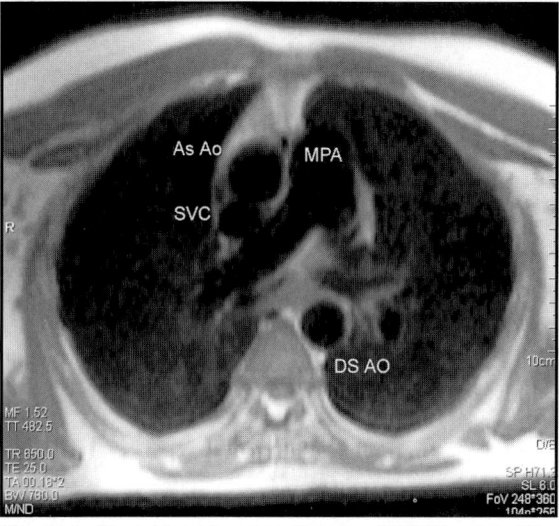

Fig. 11.1: Black blood imaging. This is a HASTE axial of the chest, which is spin-echo sequence. Note all the vessels are dark

to whole body. Therefore, a flowing nucleus that receives an excitation pulse is rephased regardless of its slice position and produces a signal. Moreover, short TR is used in GRE sequences, which results in repeated RF pulses saturating stationary tissues. This increases contrast between flowing blood and stationary tissue thus makes GRE more flow sensitive.

TYPES OF MR ANGIOGRAPHY

Basic two types of MR angiography are used in routine practice.
1. Time of flight MRA (TOF-MRA)
2. Phase contrast MRA (PC-MRA)

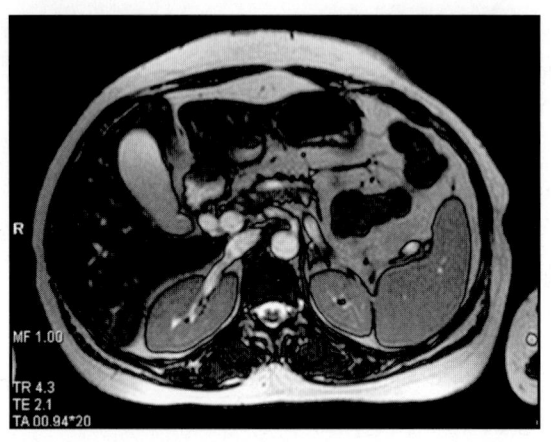

Fig. 11.2: Bright blood imaging. This is TRUFI axial image of abdomen. Trufi is a gradient echo sequence. Note aorta and other vessels are bright

Time of Flight MRA (TOF-MRA)

Time of Flight Phenomenon

To produce a signal, a nucleus must receive both excitation pulse and rephasing pulse. Stationary nuclei always receive both these pulses but flowing nuclei present in excited slice may have exited the slice before rephasing pulse hits them. This is called time of flight phenomenon. Effect of TOF phenomenon will be different in spin-echo and GRE sequences. In SE sequence TOF will result in signal void. TOF will cause flow enhancement with bright signal from flowing blood in GRE (see bright blood imaging).

The sequence used in routine practice TOF-MRA is a GRE- FLASH with gradient moment rephasing (see flash in chapter on sequences). In TOF- MRA vascular contrast is produced by manipulating LM of stationary tissues. TR is kept less than T1 of stationary tissue. This saturates (beats down) stationary spins, reducing signal from them.

Gradient moment rephasing: Nuclei flowing along a gradient will change their phase because magnetic field strength is altered along a gradient. If phase of the flowing nuclei is not maintained then signal will be altered from flowing spins. To prevent this, gradients are adjusted in such a way that spins will not lose their phase and gain phase. This is called as gradient moment repahsing or nulling (GMR).

For evaluation of arteries, spins or flowing nuclei in the veins should be nulled or saturated. This is done by applying saturation pulses in the direction of venous flow. For example, for carotid MRA, saturation pulses are applied superior to the imaging volume.

Problems with TOF MRA are flow saturation and T1 sensitivity. Spins may get saturated or beaten down as they pass down the stream in the imaging volume because they receive multiple RF pulses. This is more so if vessel runs in the plane of slice or slab. This results in reduced signal from the vessel. Because of the sensitivity of this sequence to the short T1 tissues, bright signal from these tissues like fat may interfere with vascular signal. Blood components with short T1 recovery time such as methhemoglobin also appear bright on TOF-MRA and can make differentiation of subacute hemorrhage difficult from flowing blood.

TOF-MRA can be of three types:
1. 2D TOF
2. 3D TOF
3. MOTSA (Multiple Overlapping Thin Slab Acquisitions)

In 2D TOF, acquisition is slice by slice. 2D TOF is sensitive to slow flow and gives large area of coverage. Hence it is used for slower velocity vessels like peripheral arteries and for venography. Resolution of 2D TOF is lower than that of 3D TOF.

In 3D TOF, acquisition is from whole volume of the tissue. It gives good resolution and smaller vessels are better visualised. It is usually used for high velocity flow. In 3D TOF there is a higher risk of saturating signals from spins within the volume.

MOTSA combines advantages of 2D (larger area of coverage) and 3D (high resolution). In this imaging volume is divided into multiple thin overlapping slabs during acquisition. These slabs are then combined to single volume of data (Figs 11.3 and 11.4).

Reformation of angiography: Data from TOF MRA is reformatted by technique called MIP (Maximum Intensity Projection) to get angiogram. In MIP, pixels with maximum intensity are selected and rest pixels are suppressed such that only vessels are visualised because they have pixels with maximum intensity. Disadvantage of this technique is overestimation of stenosis of vessels. Hence, viewing of source images (axial images) is always recommended before commenting on stenosis.

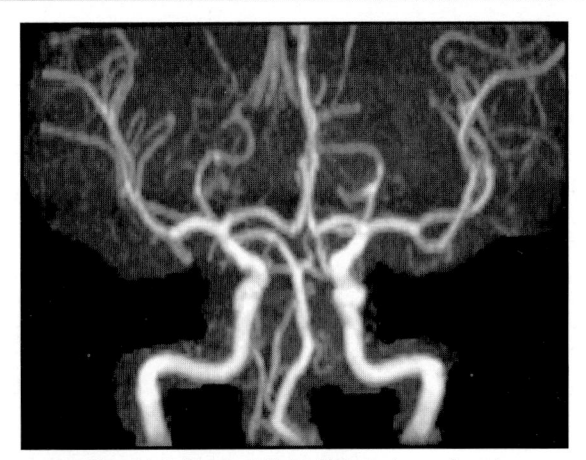

Fig. 11.3: Time of flight MR angiography of intracranial arteries

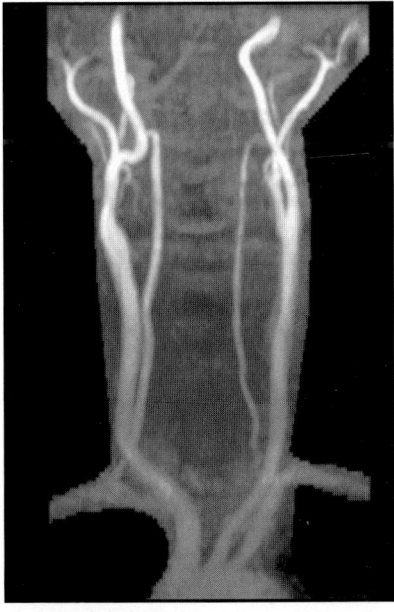

Fig. 11.4: Time of flight MR angiography of carotid and vertebral arteries

Phase Contrast MRA

PC-MRA uses changes in the phase of TM of the flowing blood to produce image contrast in flowing blood. Phase shift is selectively introduced for moving spins with use of magnetic field gradients.

After RF excitation pulse, spins are in phase. Gradients of given strength is then applied to both stationary and flowing spins. Phase shift occurs in both stationary and flowing spins, but at different rates. A second gradient pulse of same amplitude and duration but of opposite polarity is applied. In stationary nuclei reversal of phase shift occurs of exact amount, canceling the effect of original phase shift and resulting in no net phase shift. However, since flowing nuclei have changed their position, the phase shift will not be corrected. This phase shift is directly proportional to the change in location or distance the nuclei traveled between applications of first and second gradient. These phase shifts are used by PC-MRA to create angiographic images and measure flow velocities.

To provide quantitative information velocity encoding gradients are applied in one or all three directions. Velocity encoding technique compensates for projected flow velocity within the vessel by controlling the amplitude or strength of bipolar gradient. If velocity encoding (VENC) is selected lower than the velocity within the vessel, aliasing occurs. Aliasing results in low signal intensity in the center of the vessel and better delineation of vessel wall. Typical values used for VENC are-

20-30 cm/s for venous flow

MR ANGIOGRAPHY

40-60 cm/s for higher velocity with some aliasing

60-80 cm/s to determine velocity and flow direction

PC-MRA also provides information about flow direction. If flow is encoded from superior to inferior, flow from head appears bright whereas flow from feet appears black.

PC-MRA can be in 2D or 3D acquisition. 2D is more commonly used in routine practice because of its acceptable acquisition time of 1-3 minutes.

Time of Flight MRA	vs	*Phase contrast*
Uses movement of LM of blood to produce image contrast	1.	Uses movement of TM to produce contrast for the image
Less effective with slow flow because of progressive saturation	2.	PC-MRA is good for slow flow because there is no saturation.
Vessel flowing in the plane of slice show saturation hence poor signal from them.	3.	No in-plane saturation, therefore, sensitive to flow within FOV.
Takes shorter time than PCMRA	4.	PC-MRA takes longer time than TOF
Useful for rapid blood flow like extracranial carotids	5.	Useful for studying small tortuous intracranial arteries and veins, specially when blood flow is slow and in-plane.
Less sensitive to turbulence	6.	More sensitive to turbulance
Sensitive to T1 effects hence intravascular contrast media like Gadolinium can be given.	7.	Gadolinium cannot be used with phase contrast

CONTRAST ENHANCED MRA (CEMRA)

MRA also can be obtained by injecting initravascular gadolinium. Sequence used is T1-weighted 3D spoiled gradient refocused GRE sequence. Approximate T1 times of blood, muscle and enhanced blood are 1200 ms, 600 ms and 100 ms respectively. A dose of at least 0.2 mmol/kg of gadolinium is required to make T1 of blood shorter than that of fat and muscle, so that it will appear brighter than fat. However, usually double-dose gadolinium is used with 3D spoiled gradient refocused GRE sequence for CEMRA. The important issue in CEMRA is timing of peak arterial enhancement such that it will fill center of the k-space that is responsible for contrast in the image.

APPLICATIONS OF MRA

MRA has become part of management of cardiovascular and neurovascular diseases.

TOF-MRA of carotid arteries and circle of Willis are used in imaging the patients with stroke. This saves patient from radiation and contrast medium and risks of invasive procedures. In cerebral venous sinus thrombosis, phase contrast MR venography (Fig. 11.5) gives accurate diagnosis and the extent of the disease apart from parenchymal changes associated with it.

MR angiographies performed in body and the peripheral vessels are usually contrast enhanced. Body angiogram indications include aortic aneurysm, renal artery stenosis, aortoarteritis. Peripheral MR angiographies

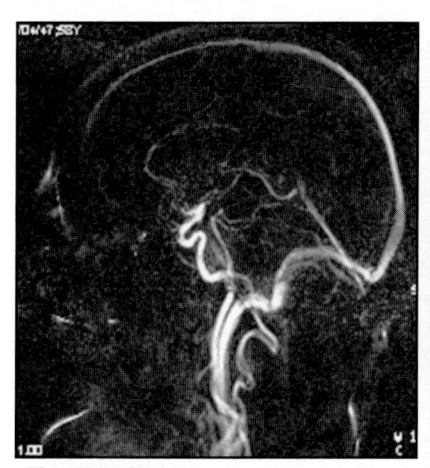

Fig. 11.5: Phase-contrast venography of intracranial venous system, sagittal view

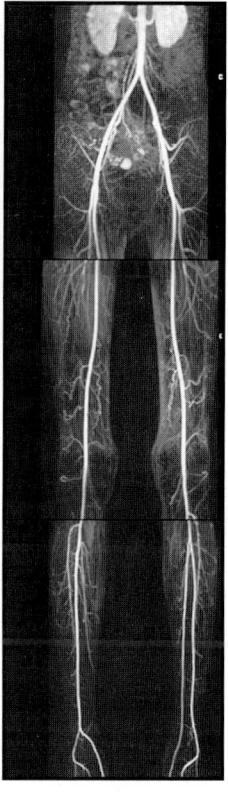

Fig. 11.6: Contrast enhanced MR angiography (CEMRA) of lower limb arteries

(Fig. 11.6) are usually performed for peripheral vascular disease, atheroscerotic arterial disease. CEMRA are specially useful in patients with compromised renal function and those with history of severe allergy to iodinated contrast media.

CHAPTER 12
MR Diffusion

INTRODUCTION

Diffusion weighted imaging is a relatively new technique in MRI that is found to be very useful in many pathologies. It forms the integral part of brain imaging protocols.

What is diffusion?

Diffusion is random movement of water protons. The process by which water protons diffuse randomly in space is called as *Brownian motion*. It is result of the dissipation of the thermal energy.

In **Isotrophic** diffusion possibility of a water protons moving in any one particular direction is equal to the probability that it will move in any other direction.

In **Anisotrophic** diffusion water diffusion has preferred direction. Water protons move more easily in some direction.

How do we acquire diffusion weighted images?

The basic sequence is called "Stesjkal-Tanner pulsed gradient spin echo sequence". It is a spin echo sequence with diffusion gradients applied before and after 180 degree pulse (Fig. 12.1).

Diffusion sequences in present use are diffusion gradient applied to echoplanar (EPI) sequence with infinite T2.

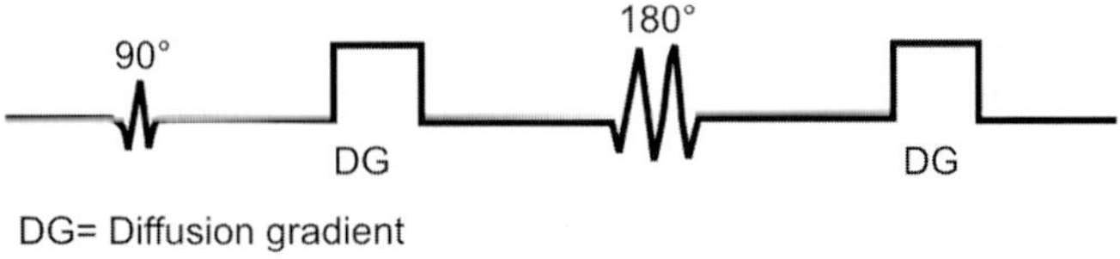

DG= Diffusion gradient

Fig. 12.1: Diagram of 'Stesjkal-Tanner' sequence

MR DIFFUSION | 173

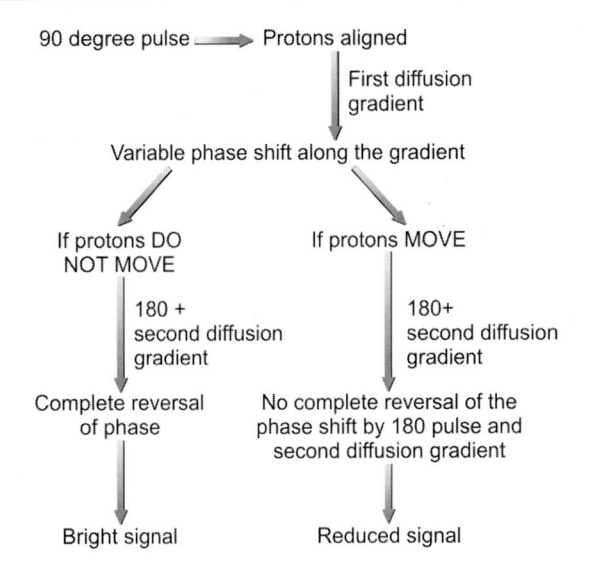

```
90 degree pulse ──▶ Protons aligned
                         │
                    First diffusion
                    gradient
                         ▼
        Variable phase shift along the gradient
         ╱                              ╲
   If protons DO                   If protons MOVE
   NOT MOVE
       │                                  │
    180 +                              180+
    second diffusion                   second diffusion
    gradient                           gradient
       ▼                                  ▼
   Complete reversal            No complete reversal of the
   of phase                     phase shift by 180 pulse and
                                second diffusion gradient
       │                                  │
       ▼                                  ▼
   Bright signal                    Reduced signal
```

Few terms and concepts need to be discussed now. They are b-value, ADC, T2 shine through and diffusion trace.

b-value

b-value indicates the magnitude of diffusion weighting provided by diffusion gradients. It also indicates sensitivity of the sequence to diffusion. It is expressed in sec/cm square. It depends on amplitude, separation and duration of diffusion gradient. B-value increases with diffusion gradient strength, duration of their application and time between applications of two gradients.

ADC: Apparent Diffusion Coefficient

Apparent diffusion coefficient is measure of diffusion. It is calculated mathematically from b-value zero and various higher b-value images. Images of ADC are called 'ADC Map'. Area with reduced ADC (restricted diffusion) will manifest as bright area on diffusion weighted images (DWI) while same area will turn dark on ADC map.

In routine practice, three sets of images are acquired. One with b-value zero (i.e. without diffusion gradients applied), second with higher b-value usually b=1000 and third set of images is automatically calculated from these two images, called as ADC map (Figs 12.2A to C). Acquisition of all three sets of images of whole brain on newer machines and with EPI technique takes 40-45 seconds.

T2 Shine Through

Signal intensity on DWI not only depends on ADC but also on tissue T2. This T2 can cause paradoxical decrease in signals of restricted diffusion or when diffusion is normal can be mistaken for restricted diffusion on DWI. To differentiate this T2 shine through from actual restricted diffusion, ADC maps are used. ADC map will show reduced signal in actually diffusion restricted area while there will be bright signal in case of T2 shine through on ADC map.

Diffusion "Trace"

To average out anisotrophic white matter tract effects on diffusion of water, image with higher b-value like b=1000

MR DIFFUSION 175

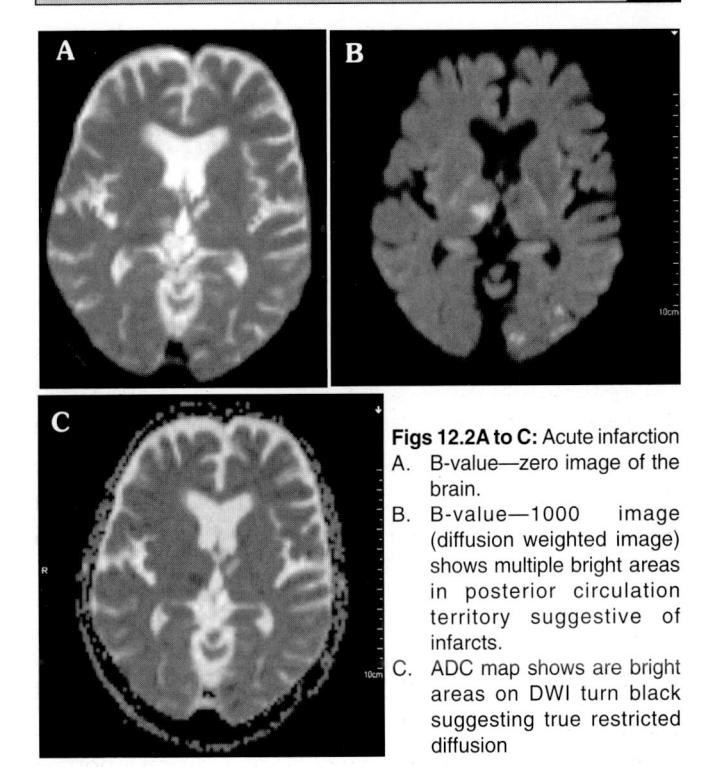

Figs 12.2A to C: Acute infarction
A. B-value—zero image of the brain.
B. B-value—1000 image (diffusion weighted image) shows multiple bright areas in posterior circulation territory suggestive of infarcts.
C. ADC map shows are bright areas on DWI turn black suggesting true restricted diffusion

is taken in three directions—X, Y, Z axes. Diffusion changes along all three axes then averaged to get image called 'trace' diffusion image.

CLINICAL USES OF DIFFUSION

Stroke

In ischemia there is failure of Na-K ATPase pump, which results into influx of water into the cells. This is called as cytotoxic edema. Since there is net shift of water molecules

176 MRI MADE EASY (FOR BEGINNERS)

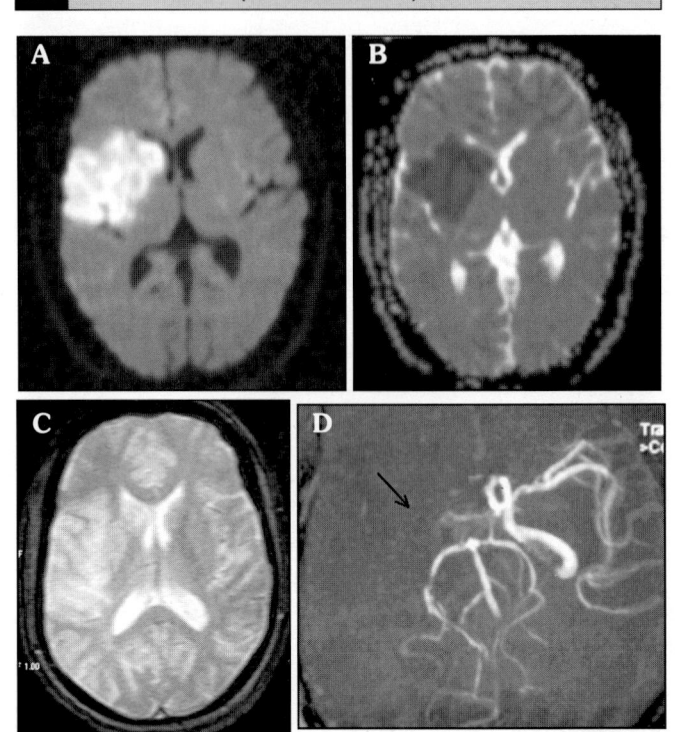

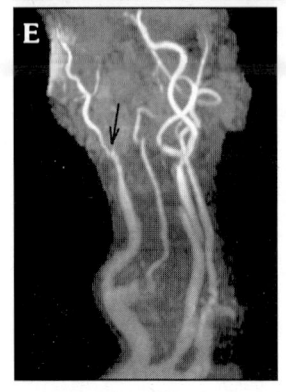

Figs 12.3A to E: A typical case of stroke.
A. DWI shows bright area in the right parietal region.
B. On ADC map image the area turns black suggestive of acute infarct.
C. On gradient Hemo image no evidence of any bleeding, making the infarct non-hemorrhagic
D. TOF MRA of Circle of Willis shows absent right ICA, MCA and ACA (arrow).
E. TOR MRA of carotid arteries shows complete occlusion of right ICA from its origin (arrow).

from extracellular into more restricted intracellular space, there is overall reduction in diffusion of water in that area. This will be manifested as bright signal on DWI and dark signals on ADC map. So diffusion imaging can detect early ischaemic tissue as early as minutes to hours. DWI shows stroke lesion when all other images including T2-weighted images are normal (Figs 12.3A to E). It takes CBF to drop below 15-20 ml/100 gm of brain tissue /minute to be manifested as bright signal on DWI (reduced ADC).

As against cytotoxic edema, vasogenic edema, which is increased fluid in extracellular space, will show increased diffusion (increased ADC). Chronic infarct is dark on DWI and bright on ADC (Figs 12.4A and B).

Hypoxic Ischemic Injury to Newborns

Cytotoxic edema is easily appreciated on DWI in HIE in newborns. Regions commonly affected include basal ganglion and water-shed areas.

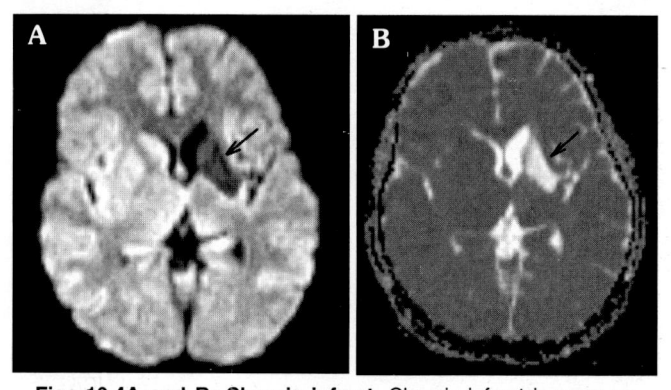

Figs 12.4A and B: Chronic infarct. Chronic infarct is seen as hypointense on DWI (A) and bright on ADC map (B)

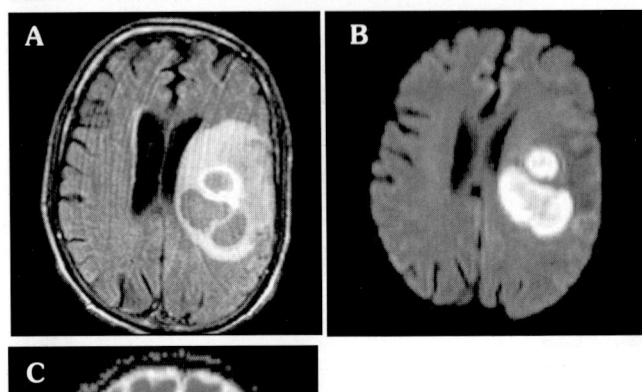

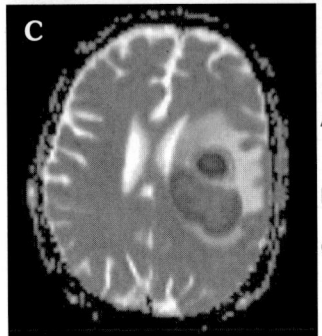

Figs 12.5A to C: Abscess
A. FLAIR image shows a large abscess in left cerebral hemisphere
B. DWI shows central part of the abscess to be bright
C. On ADC map the central part of the abscess turns black suggestive of restricted diffusion

Epidermoid versus Arachnoid Cyst

Epidermoid is composed of keratin, debries and solid cholesterol, which provide barrier or hindrance to water proton diffusion. This results into epidermoid to be bright on DWI. Since arachnoid cyst is a clear CSF containing cyst, it will be same as CSF signal intensity.

Abscess versus Cystic Neoplasm

Abscess contains thick fluid with hindrances to water diffusion. Hence it shows restricted diffusion (bright on DWI) in the center. Neoplasm with central necrosis does not show restricted diffusion in the center (Figs 12.5A to C).

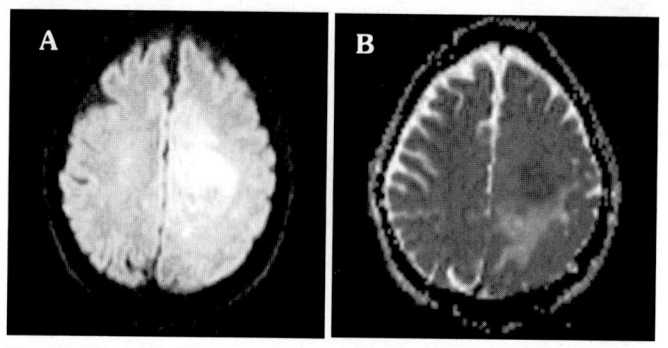

Figs 12.6A and B: This is a case of lymphoma in left cerebral hemisphere which is bright on DWI (A) and dark on ADC (B) suggesting restricted diffusion of water molecules due to high cellularity

Lymphoma versus Toxoplasma in HIV

Ratio of ADC in the center of rim enhancing intra-cranial lesion relative to normal white matter is significantly higher in Toxoplasmosis. ADC ratio more than 1.6 is only seen in toxoplasmosis and ADC ratio less than one is seen only in lymphoma (Figs 12.6A and B).

Diffusion on Posttreatment Assessment

DWI detects residual epidermoid. In chemotherapy there is sharp increase in ADC within first two weeks of treatment. Increase in ADC corresponds with volume of tissue killed. This is of prognostic value.

DIFFUSION TENSOR

Routine diffusion weighted imaging is done for isotrophic diffusion. Tensor diffusion is done for anisotrophic diffusion.

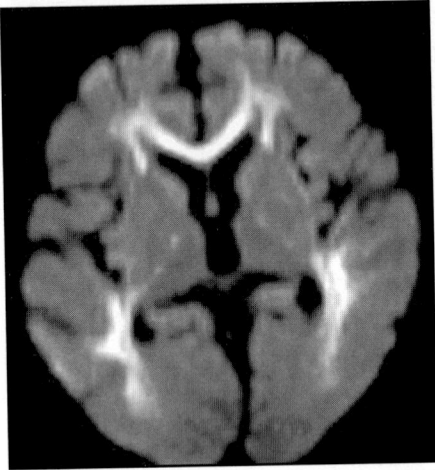

Fig. 12.7: DWI image (fractional analysis image) in one direction (anterior to posterior) shows bright genu and optic radiations because these fibres are perpendicular in this direction. Such images in 12 or 24 directions are taken to get the tractography

Tensor is the mathematical formalism used to model anisotrophic diffusion.

Technique

MR scanner axes—X,Y, Z are never perfectly parallel to white matter tract at every point in the image. Hence images are acquired in multiple directions- six or twelve, instead of three in usual trace diffusion (Fig. 12.7). From these images in multiple directions pure apparent diffusion coefficient for each pixel is calculated. This is called as *'principal eigen value'*. Principal eigen value is calculated along the true axis of diffusion called as *'eigen vector'*. The image formed with principal eigen value is called as diffusion tensor image.

Uses: Diffusion tensor measures the magnitude of the ADC in the preferred direction of water diffusion and also perpendicular to the direction. The resultant image shows white matter tracts very well. Hence this technique also called as 'tractography'. Tractography is useful for relationship of tracts with tumor, tumor invasion of tracts and preoperative planning.

CHAPTER 13

MR Perfusion

INTRODUCTION

Perfusion refers to the passage of blood from an arterial supply to venous drainage through the microcirculation. Perfusion is necessary for the nutritive supply to tissues and for clearance of products of metabolism. Perfusion gets changed by various pathologies affecting the particular tissue. Hence measuring changes in perfusion can be helpful in diagnosis of diseases, monitoring and assessing treatment response.

Blood flow and metabolism of human tissues have been studied with tracers for many years and now with positron emission tomography (PET). These techniques lack spatial and temporal resolution as well as specificity. Radiological methods include CT perfusion and MR perfusion. MR perfusion can be performed with exogenous (injectable) contrast agent like Gadolinium or by endogenous contrast agent. In this chapter we will mainly discuss MR perfusion with injectable contrast and its clinical applications. We will also discuss in short, basic principles of endogenous methods like arterial spin labeling (ASL).

MR Perfusion with Exogenous Contrast Agent

Technique

0.2 mmol/kg of Gd-DTPA is injected intravenously at the rate of 5 ml/second and rapid $T2^*$-weighted EPI sequence is run for 60-90 seconds. Multiple measurements are taken as Gd passes through the circulation.

Mechanism

Paramagnetic agents like Gd cause shortening of both T1 and T2 of the tissue or region in which they go. Decrease in T1 relaxation time on T1-weighted images results into increased signals or brightening. Reduction in T2 relaxation time on T2 or T2*-weighted images results into signal drop or blackening (Table 13.1). In perfusion as gadolinium passes through the microvasculature there is decrease in signal from magnetic susceptibility induced shortening of T2* relaxation times. So more the signal drop more will be the perfusion. Considering concentration of contrast agent constant, more the number of small vessels per voxel of tissue, more will be signal drop. Thus, microvascularity or relative perfusion of that region or tissue can be determined.

Parameters

From the raw data images thus acquired various colour-coded maps are constructed. These are relative maps in that the arterial input function is not typically measured and hence true quantitative volumes (ml blood/gm tissue/time) are not routinely calculated.

rCBV: Relative cerebral blood volume
CBF : Cerebral blood flow
TTP : Time to peak
MTT : Mean transit time

Permiability/Leakiness

Areas of severe blood-brain barrier break-down are frequently seen in necrotic tumor and irradiated tumor beds. Increased permiability or leakiness because of break in blood-brain barrier results in Gd in extravascular space. T1- enhancing effects of this Gd may predominate to counteract the T2 signal lowering effects of Gd, resulting in falsely low rCBV values. Measures to reduce the permeability induced effects on rCBV include mathematical correction with calculation of permiability or K2 maps (Fig. 13.1) and use of Dysprosium that has stronger T2* effects but negligible T1 effects, instead of Gd.

Table 13.1: Routine contrast enhancement versus perfusion imaging

	Routine contrast enhancement	*Perfusion imaging*
1. Sequence	T1-weighted imaging	T2*-weighted EPI sequence
2. Signal change	Increase in signal intensity	Drop in signal intensity
3. Mechanism	Gd caused reduction in T1 relaxation time.	Gd caused reduction in T2 or T2* relaxation time and magnetic susceptibility
4. Detects	Break in blood-brain barrier leading to leakage of Gd	Gd in microvasculature (capillaries). Thus gives information about amount of small vessels (vascularity) and perfusion of the tissue.

Clinical Applications

MR perfusion has been studied for clinical utility in various conditions like stroke, brain tumors, dementia and

MR PERFUSION 187

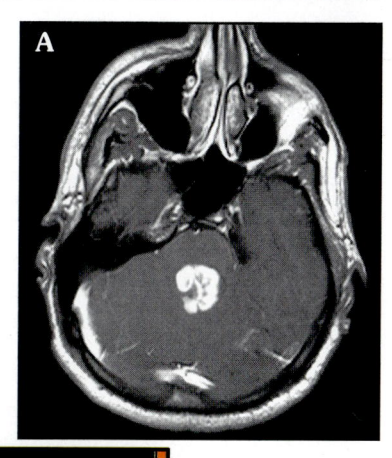

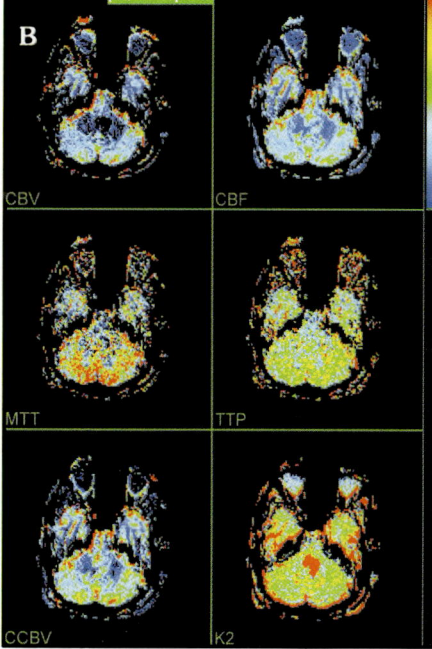

Fig. 13.1: Permiability map
A. Enhancing tumor is seen in the pons.
B. Perfusion maps- On CBV map the lesion is hypovascular (dark) but when K2 map (permeability map) is calculated and corrected CBV (CCBV) is calculated the lesion is hypervascular (red). Redness of the lesion on K2 map is because of increased permeability due to break in blood brain barrier (last image)

psychiatric illnesses, migraine headaches, trauma, epilepsy and multiple sclerosis. We will discuss its role in stroke and tumors, where it is commonly used in clinical practice.

MR Perfusion in Stroke

With concept of stroke as 'brain attack' and availability and acceptance for thrombolytic agents, it becomes very important to detect brain ischemia and salvageable tissue in early window period of 3-6 hours. DWI (diffusion weighted imaging) and PWI (perfusion weighted imaging) together are very effective in detection of early ischaemia long before infarction or any abnormality seen on T2-weighted images. Mismatch between PW and DW represent potentially salvageable tissue (penumbra) (Fig. 13.2).

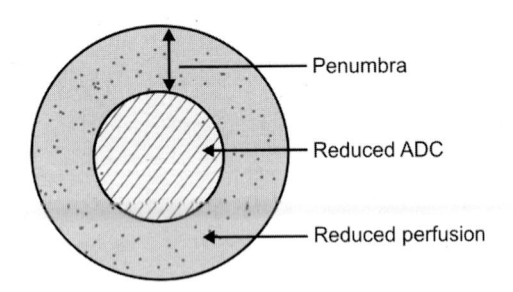

Fig. 13.2: Penumbra

PW-DW mismatch is also indicator of clinical outcome. Small mismatch has good clinical outcome. Large mismatch is associated with poor clinical outcome and larger vessel occlusion.

PWI is more sensitive than DWI for detecting ischemia in early period after the onset of arterial occlusion. Restricted diffusion (reduced ADC) always accompanied by total or near total perfusion deficit and there appears to be a threshold in humans before tissue becomes abnormal on DWI, despite low rCBV. If decrease in perfusion is mild ADC may be normal.

Presence of perfusion delay (raised MTT/raised TTP) is considered to represent tissue at risk whereas decreased ADC represents metabolic jeopardy.

MR Perfusion in Brain Tumors

Gliomas—MR Perfusion is useful in grading gliomas, in guiding biopsies and differentiating therapy induced necrosis from recurrent/residual tumor.

It has been shown that rCBV correlates with both conventional angiographic assessment of tumor vascularity and histologic measurement of tumor neovascularity. rCBV is surrogate marker of tumor angiogenesis and malignancy, and statistically significant correlation has been found between rCBV and glioma grading (Figs 13.3A to D).

rCBV helps to guide biopsies. Tumor area with highest rCBV value yields good results and increases diagnostic confidence.

RCBV maps can differentiate between therapy induced necrosis (decreased rCBV/ complete loss of rCBV) from recurrent/residual tumor (elevated rCBV) (Figs 13.4A to D).

Metastasis—Perfusion may help in differentiating a solitary metastasis from glioma based on differences in measurement of peritumoral rCBV. In metastasis, there is no histological evidence of tumor beyond the outer contrast enhancing margin of the tumor so rCBV will not be raised. In high grade glioma, the peritumoral region represents

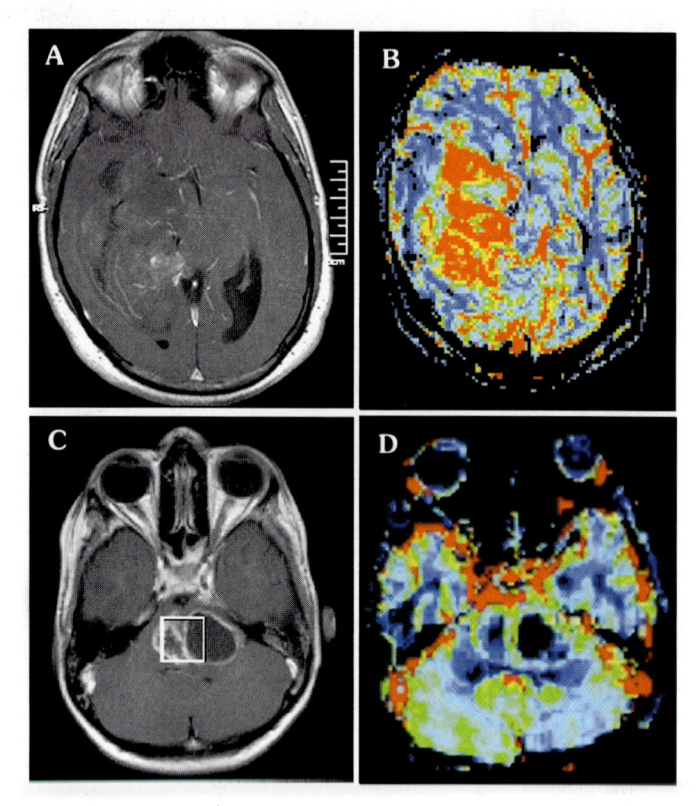

Figs 13.3A to D: High grade versus low grade glioma
A. Post-contrast T1-w axial image of the brain shows Nonenhancing tumor in the right cerebral hemisphere
B. CCBV map shows the tumor to be hypervascular (red) suggestive of high grade tumor
C. Post-contrast T1-w axial image of the brain shows cystic solid lesion in the pons
D. On perfusion the lesion is hypovascular suggestive of low grade tumor

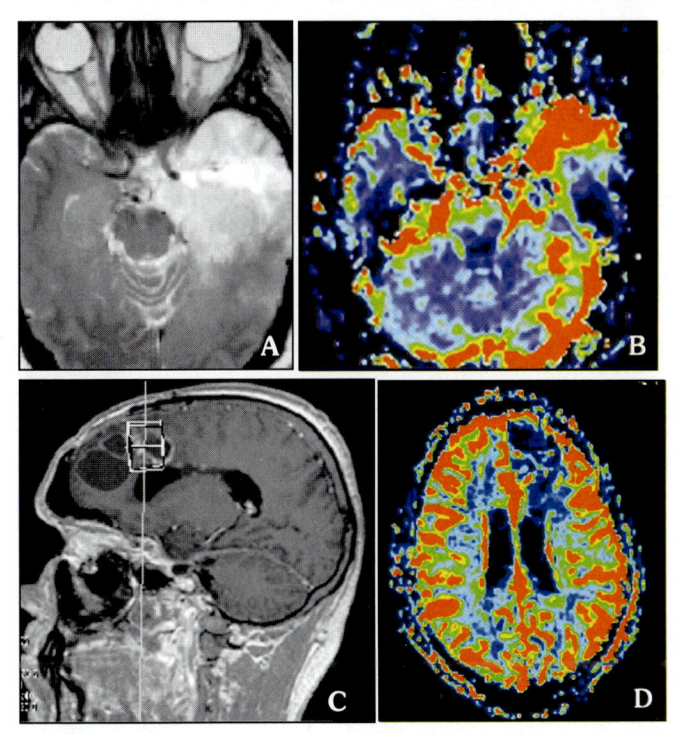

Figs 13.4A to D: Recurrence versus necrosis
A. Postradiation tumor in the left temporal lobe
B. The tumor in (A) is hypervascular on CCBV (red) map suggesting recurrence
C. Postoperative, post radiation tumor in the left frontal lobe
D. The tumor in (C) is hypovascular suggesting radiation necrosis

a variable combination of vesogenic edema and tumor cells infiltrating along perivascular spaces hence shows increased rCBV.

Lymphoma, medulloblastoma have high cellularity with high nuclear-cytoplasmic ratio hence show reduced rCBV.

Neoplasms like oligodendroglioma, meningioma and vascular metastases from renal cell carcinoma and melanoma show increased rCBV. However, meningioma may show falsely high or falsely low rCBV. This is because meningioma lack blood-brain barrier that results into immediate contrast leakage of contrast without any substantial recovery of T2* signal loss back to baseline.

Differentiation of neoplasm from tumor mimicking lesions- perfusion may differentiate tumor from infection, infarction, tumefactive demyelinating lesion (TDL). Histologically TDL consists of perivascular inflammatory infiltration and demyelination. Hypervascularity is rare in this lesion. TDL can be difficult to differentiate from tumors not only radiologically but also histologically. There is absence of frank neoangiogenesis in TDL. Hence perfusion will not show raised rCBV in TDL.

Other Clinical Uses

MR perfusion is also used to assess ischaemic or hypoperfused areas in conditions like Moyamoya disease (Fig. 13.5), CNS vasculitis.

ARTERIAL SPIN LABELING (ASL)

ASL is a non-invasive method to assess tissue perfusion without exogenous contrast injection or radiation.

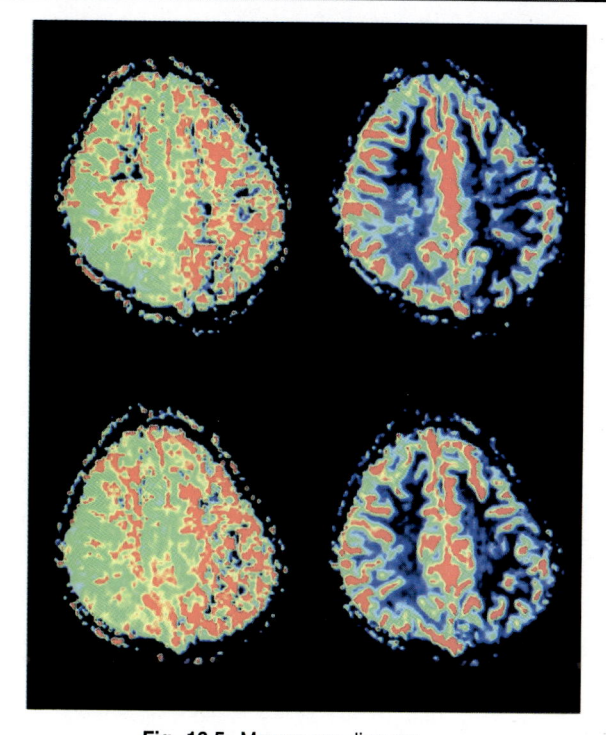

Fig. 13.5: Moyamoya disease

MTT maps (left side images) show increased MTT in left cerebral hemisphere.

CBV map (right side images) show reduced CBV in the left cerebral hemisphere.

This is suggestive of perfusion compromise (reduction) in the left cerebral hemisphere

ASL is done as follows (Fig. 13.6)

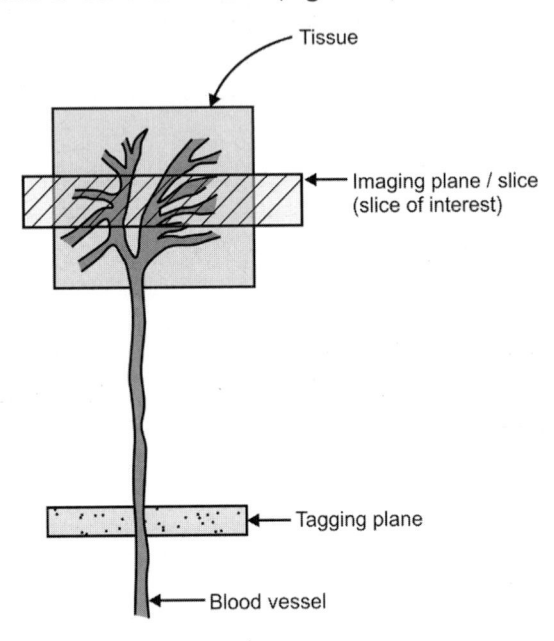

Fig. 13.6: Arterial spin labelling (diagram)

Arterial blood flowing towards the region of interest is tagged by magnetic inversion pulses (proton phase is changed).

↓

After a delay to allow for inflow of tagged blood, image is acquired in slice of interest. This image is called 'tag image'.

↓

Second image of same slice of interest is again

acquired without in-flowing tagged blood. This image is called 'control image'.

↓

Tag image is subtracted from control image.

↓

This results into perfusion image representing 'tagged blood' that flowed into the image slice.

ASL involves T1- weighted imaging.

It has poor SNR, however, ASL has better spatial and temporal resolution than PET. Poor SNR and sensitivity to abnormally long transit delays of tagged protons prevents its general application.

CHAPTER 14

MR Spectroscopy

INTRODUCTION

MR Spectroscopy (MRS) is an exciting application of magnetic resonance to access various metabolites or biochemical from the body tissues non-invasively. This metabolite information is then used to diagnose diseases, monitoring the diseases and assessing response to the treatment. Even though theorotically MRS can be performed with spins or nuclei of 1H, 13C, 19F, 23Na, 31P, MRS in present clinical use are mainly 1H (Hydrogen) and 31P (Phosphorus) spectroscopy. Discussion in this chapter mainly relates to 1H or Proton spectroscopy because of its widespread use.

The basic principles of MRS are same as magnetic resonance imaging (MRI). However, few differences exist.

1. MR images are reconstructed from the entire proton signal from the tissue dominated by water and fat proton signals. Protons from other metabolites do not contribute to imaging because of their negligible concentration.

    As against MRI, the aim in MRS itself is to detect these small metabolites. Most metabolite signals of clinical interest resonate between resonant frequencies of water and fat. To be able to detect these small metabolites large signal from water protons need to be suppressed.

2. How are small metabolites from the tissue detected? Chemical shift forms the basis of MRS, while it is one of causes of artifacts in MRI.

Precessional frequency of protons is determined by the chemical environment or electron cloud surrounding it. Proton in water will precess at different frequency than proton in fat, and the same proton in other metabolite for example NAA will precess at different frequency than in water and fat. This change in precessional frequency of protons because of different chemical environment is *chemical shift*. So by determining the frequency of protons we can detect their chemical environment, i.e. metabolites in which they are precessing.

In a homogeneous field,

Frequency of protons in a given metabolites = chemical shift = position of metabolite peak.

Since the precessional frequency of any proton is directly proportional to the external magnetic field strength (Larmor frequency), chemical shift in Hz will be different at different magnetic field strength. To avoid this confusion chemical shift is expressed in parts per million (ppm), which will be same for a particular metabolite at all field strengths.

Since chemical shift is proportional to external magnetic field, smaller chemical shift will not be detected at low field strength. Even though MRS can be performed on 0.5 Tesla or above, field strength of 1.5 T or above are required for improved spectral separation and increased SNR.

3. Magnetic Field Homogeneity

Magnetic field should be homogeneous, i.e. of same

strength throughout its entire extent for all MR applications. MRS requires much more homogeneous field than MRI because the smaller concentrations of metabolites with smaller chemical shift needs to be detected. Since chemical shift is proportional to external magnetic field, smaller chemical shift will be misinterpreted and incorrect concentration will be recorded in inhomogeneous field.

Homogeneity required for MRI is about 1 to 10 ppm while for MRS it is about 0.1 ppm.

The process of making the magnetic field homogeneous is called as *shimming*.

4. No frequency encoding gradient in MRS

    As in MRI, localization in MRS is done by slice selection and phase encoding gradient. However, frequency encoding gradient is not used in MRS to preserve optimal homogeneity and chemical shift information.

    One more phenomenon needs to be discussed in MRS is *spin-spin or J-coupling*. Spins (protons) with small difference of precessional frequency for example spins within a molecule interact with each other. This is facilitated by electrons around the nuclei. This spin-spin interaction modifies the resonant frequency of a spin involved in it. J-coupling causes fusion of peaks on spectral map, e.g. doublet of lactate at 1.3 ppm.

Localization Techniques in MRS

In initial days, localisation of the volume of interest from which metabolite information is obtained, was done by

MR SPECTROSCOPY

surface coil. Area (volume) covered by the coil was the volume of interest from which metabolite information obtained. In present clinical practice four methods are commonly used for localisation of volume of interest. They are STEAM, PRESS, ISIS and CSI (MRSI). STEAM, PRESS and ISIS are used for single voxel spectroscopy (SVS). CSI is multivoxel (MVS) technique.

STEAM: Stimulated Echo Acquisition Method

Volume of interest is excited by three 90 degree pulses in three orthogonal planes. Since echo is stimulated signals are weak. STEAM is used in short TE (20-30 ms) spectroscopy.

PRESS: Point Resolved Spectroscopy

In PRESS, one 90 degree and two 180 degree pulses are applied along three orthogonal planes. Signals are strong and PRESS is used for longer TE (135, 270 ms) spectroscopy. PRESS can not be used for shorter TEs.

ISIS: Image Selected in vivo Spectroscopy

Three frequency selective inversion pulses are applied in presence of orthogonal gradients. Fourth non-selective pulse is used for observation of signal. ISIS is used in 31P spectroscopy.

CSI: Chemical Shift Imaging

CSI is used for multivoxel spectroscopy, where large area is covered divided into multiple voxels. CSI is also called

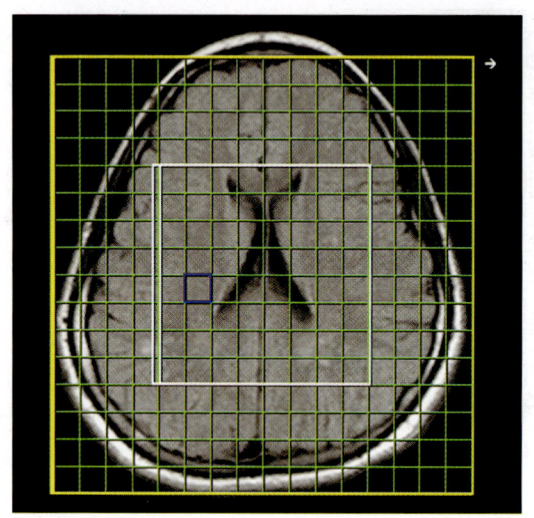

Fig. 14.1: VOI with Grid. Blue-voxel, white-volume of interest from which data is acquired and green-grid to prevent lipid contamination from the scalp interfering with signals

as Magnetic Resonance Spectroscopic Imaging (MRSI) as it combines features of both imaging and spectroscopy (Fig. 14.1). Spatial localistion is done by phase encoding in one, two or three directions to get on, two or three dimentional spectroscopy. Matabolite maps or matabolic ratio maps can be seen overlapped over the images.

Having seen the basics behind MRS, let's now go through the steps to obtain MRS:
1. Patient positioning
2. Global shimming

Optimisation of magnetic field homogeneity is done over the entire volume detected by receiver coil. Global shimming provides starting value for localized shimming.

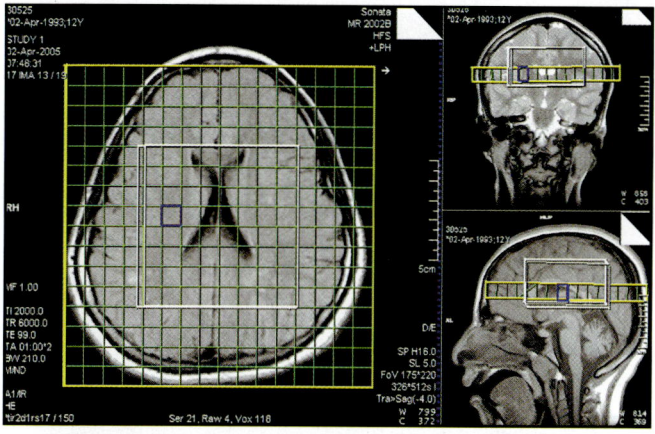

Fig. 14.2: Three planes localization of the voxel and VOI. Note position of voxel in all three planes

3. Acquisition of MR images for localization
   Images are obtained in all three planes (coronal, axial and sagittal) for placement of voxel. MR images already obtained during routine imaging can be used for the localization purpose if patient is not moved (Fig. 14.2).
4. Selection of MRS measurement and parameters
   TR and TE are important parameters. Improved SNR is obtained at longer TR.
   TEs commonly used are 20-30 ms, 135-145 ms and 270 ms (Figs 14.3A to C). At longer TEs more than 135 ms peaks of major brain metabolites only like choline, creatine, NAA and lactate are visible. Peaks from lipid, glutamate, glutamine, GABA, inositols are

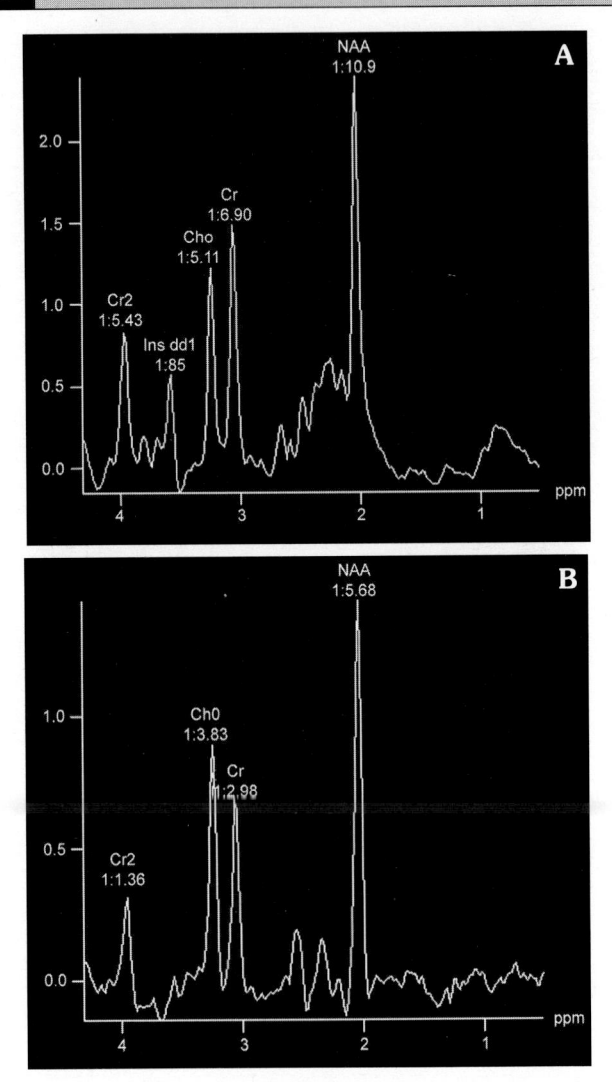

Figs 14.3A and B

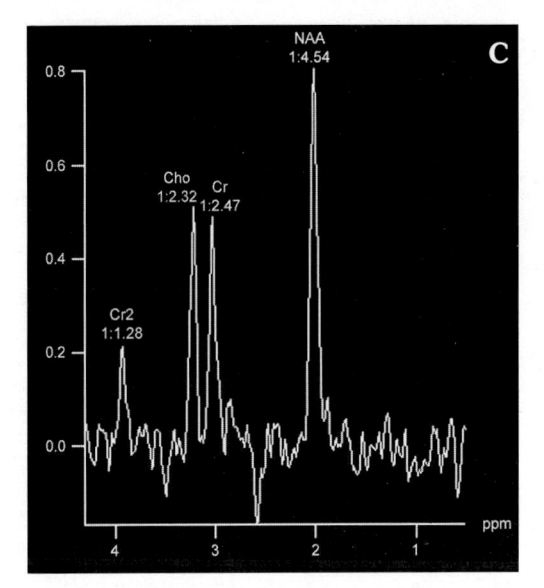

Figs 14.3A to C: Normal spectra at 30 (A), 135 (B) and 270 ms (C)

suppressed at higher TEs. There is less noise at higher TEs. Shorter TEs are used for metabolites with short T2 such as glutamate, glutamine, inositol.

5. Selection of VOI (volume of interest)

   SVS can be used for local or diffuse diseases. CSI is used in irregularly-shaped large pathology is used and where other side comparison is required (Fig. 14.4).

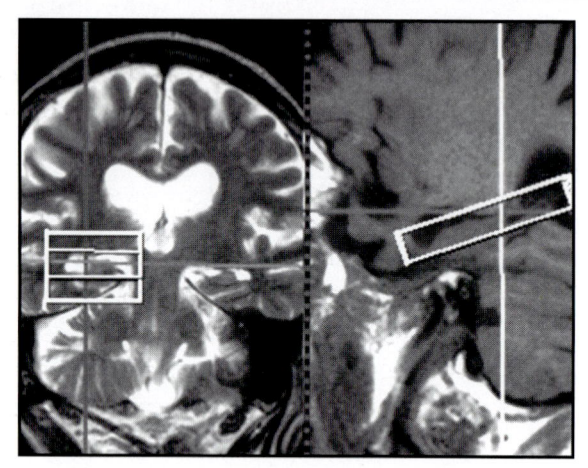

Fig. 14.4: Placement of VOI. In Alzheimer's disease hippocampus is the VOI. See the placement of VOI (white box)

6. Localized shimming

   This is optimisation of homogeneity over selected volume of interest. Good local shim results into narrower metabolite peaks, better spectral resolution and good SNR. Full width at half height of water peak is used as shim. A local shim of 4-10 Hz is desirable.

7. Water suppression

   Water peak is suppressed so that smaller metabolite peaks are visible. Water peak suppression is done by CHESS (Chemical shift selective spectroscopy) technique.

8. MRS data collection

   On modern machines in use, SVS usually takes 3-6 minutes and CSI usually takes upto 12 minutes for data acquisition.

9. Data processing and display
   Acquired data is processed to get spectrum and spectral maps. Zero point of spectrum is set in the software itself by frequency of a particular compound called Tetramethylsilane (TMS).
10. Interpretation
    Area under the peak of any metabolite is directly proportional to the number of spins contributing to the peak. Absolute values for each metabolite may vary with age and population. Interpretation should always base on ratios of metabolites and comparison with normal side.

Metabolites of 1H MRS

Table 14.1: Major metabolites

SN	Metabolites	Peak position in ppm	Approx concentration in mmol/kg in white matter
1.	NAA	2.02	10-15
2.	Creatine	3.0	8
3.	Choline	3.2	1.5
4.	Myoinositol	3.56	5

NAA: N-Acetylaspartate

Peak position: 2.02 ppm.

There is contribution from NAAG and glutamate to the NAA peak.

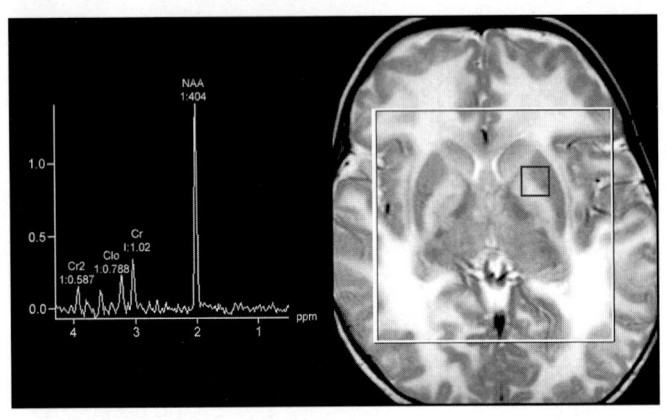

Fig. 14.5: Canavan disease. Note markedly elevated NAA peak

It is a neuronal marker and any insult to brain causing neuronal loss or degeneration causes reduction of NAA. It is absent in tissues with no neurons e.g. metastasis, meningioma.

NAA reduced in: hypoxia, infarction, Alzheimer's, Herpes encephalitis, hydrocephalus, Alexander's disease, Epilepsy, Neoplasms, stroke, NPH, Closed head trauma (Diffuse Axonal Injury).

NAA increased in: Canavan's disease (Fig. 14.5).

Cr: Creatine

Peak position: 3.0 ppm. Second peak at 3.94 ppm

The Cr peak contains contribution from creatine, CrPO4, GABA, Lysine, glutathione.

Cr serves as high energy phosphates and as a buffer in ATP/ADP reservoir. It increases with age.

Cr is increased in hypometabolic states and in trauma.

Cr is reduced in hypermetabolic states, hypoxia, stroke, tumor.

Cr remains stable in many diseases hence serves as reference or control peak for comparison.

Cho: Choline

Peak position: 3.22 ppm.

Choline is a constituent of phospholipids of cell membrane. It is precursor of acetyl choline and phosphatidyl choline. Choline is indicator of cell membrane integrity.

Cho increases with increased cell membrane synthesis and increased cell turnover.

Cho increased in: Chronic hypoxia, epilespy, Alzheimer's, gliomas and other tumors, trauma, infarction, hyperosmolar states, diabetes mellitus.

Cho reduced in: hepatic encephalopathy, stroke.

ml: Myoinositol

Peak position: 3.56 ppm. Second peak at 4.1 ppm.

MI acts as an osmolyte and is a marker of gliosis. It isinvolved in hormone sensitive neuroreception and is precursor of glucuronic acid. It is the dominant peak in newborns and decreases with age.

MI increased in: Alzheimer's, frotal lobe dementias, diabetes, hyperosmolar states.

MI decreased in: hepatic and hypoxic encephalopathy, stroke, tumor, osmotic pontine myelinolysis, hyponatremia.

Lac: Lactate

Peak position: 1.3 ppm.

It is a doublet. It is inverted at TE of 135 ms on PRESS and upright on other TEs on PRESS and at all TEs on STEAM sequences.

It is not seen in normal brain spectrum.

It is elevated in hypoxia, tumor, mitochondrial encphalopathy, IC haemorrhage, stroke, hypoventilation, Canavan's disease, Alexander, hydrocephalus.

Glx: Glutamate (Glu) and Glutamine (Gln)

Peak position: 2- 2.45 ppm for beta and gamma Glx. Second peak of alpha Glx at 3.6-3.8 ppm.

Glu is excitatory neurotransmitter and GABA is important product of Glu. Gln has role in detoxification and regulation of neurotransmitter activities.

Glx elevated in head injury, hepatic encephalopathy, hypoxia.

Lipids

Peak position: 0.9, 1.3, 1.5 ppm.

Not seen in normal brain spectrum

Seen in acute destruction of myelin.

Increased in high grade tumors (reflects necrosis), stroke, multiple sclerosis lesions and tuberculomas.

Amino Acids

Alanine (at 1.3-1.4 ppm), **Valine** (at 0.9 ppm), **leucine** (at 3.6 ppm) are usually multiplets visualised at short TE. They invert at TE of 135 ms.

Alanine is seen in meningioma whereas Valine and leucine are markers of abscess.

Glucose

Seen next to Cho peak on left side. Increased in diabetes, parenteral feeding, hepatic encephalopathy.

GABA

- 1.9 and 2.3 ppm
- Used for monitoring vigabatrin therapy.

Clinical Uses of MRS

1H (Proton) MRS has its role in almost every neurological condition. Role of MRS in few common conditions will be discussed here.

Brain Tumors

In tumors there is increase in Cho, lactate and lipid. There is reduction in NAA and Cr.

a. MRS in tumor evaluation: MRS can differentiate neoplasm from non-neoplastic lesions. MRS also helps to grade gliomas based on metabolite ratios (Figs 14.6A to C).
b. In treatment planning: MRS guides biopsy. Biopsy of higher choline area has shown higher success and

212 MRI MADE EASY (FOR BEGINNERS)

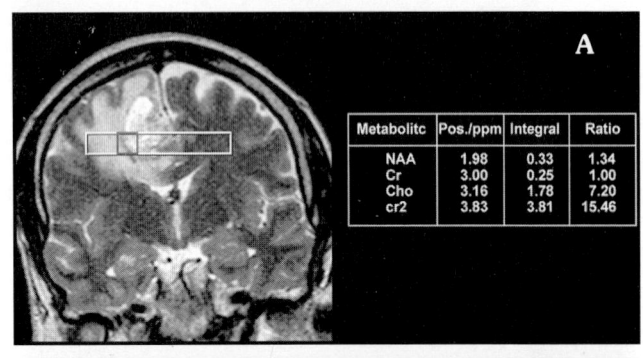

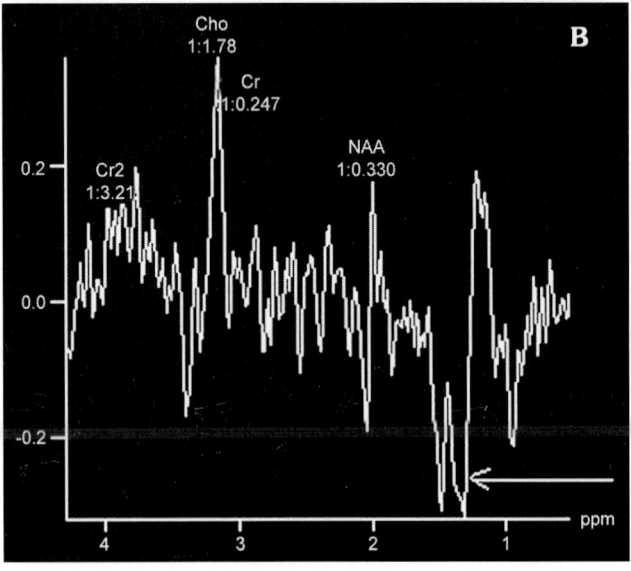

Metabolite	Pos./ppm	Integral	Ratio
NAA	1.98	0.33	1.34
Cr	3.00	0.25	1.00
Cho	3.16	1.78	7.20
cr2	3.83	3.81	15.46

Figs 14.6A and B

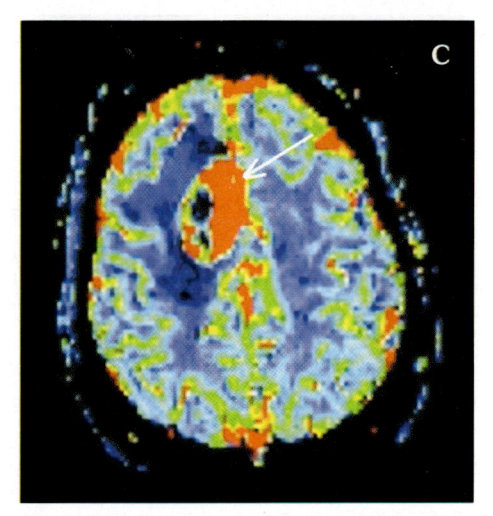

Figs 14.6A to C: High grade glioma
Tumor is seen in right parietal region (A). Note elevated choline ratio of 7.2 (in table) and elevated peak in the spectrum (B). Also seen is bifid inverted lactate peak (arrow). The tumor is hypervascular on perfusion image. All these findings are suggestive of high grade tumor

increased diagnostic confidence (Fig. 14.7). Inclusion of peritumoral area with increased cho in radiation improves survival.

In Treatment Monitoring

MRS helps to solve very important issue of differentiation of radiation necrosis and gliosis from residual or recurrent neoplasm. Patient with radiation necrosis will have reduced peaks of all metabolites whereas recurrent/residual tumor will have characteristic spectrum of tumor with elevated choline (Figs 14.8A and B).

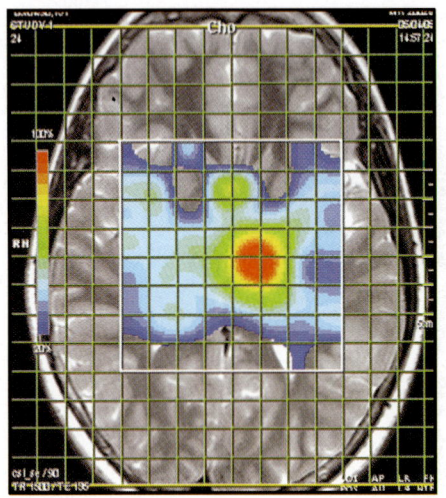

Fig. 14.7: Choline map for biopsy guidance. Biopsy from red (high choline) area yields high diagnostic results

Neonatal Hypoxia

There is decrease in NAA, Cr, MI and increase in Cho, lactate/lipid peaks in neonatal hypoxia. MRS can predict outcome of neonatal hypoxia. Progressive decrease in NAA, Cr and MI can be used to monitor the condition. In neonatal hemorrhage MRS can be used to determine hypoxia, as hypoxia is one of the causes of neonatal hemorrhage.

Metabolic Disorders and White Matter Diseases

Elevation of lactate doublet is seen in mitochondrial disorders like MELAS (Mitochondrial Encephalopathy Lactic Acidosis and Stroke) (Fig. 14.9).

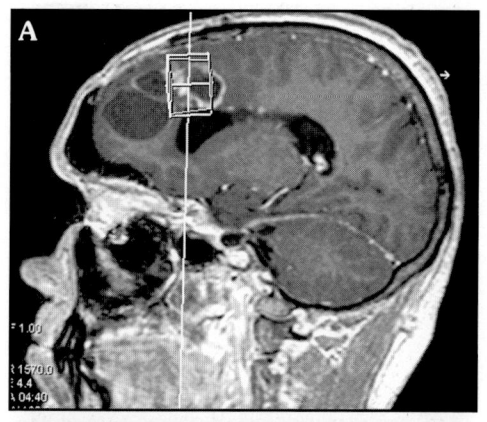

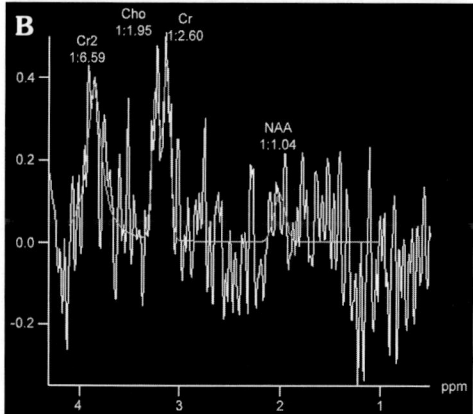

Figs 14.8A and B: Radiation necrosis.
Same patient as shown in 13.4C and D. Spectrum
(B) shows lots of noise and no dominant peak

Canavan can be differentiated easily from Alexander disease by MRS. Canavan shows elevation of NAA peak.

216 MRI MADE EASY (FOR BEGINNERS)

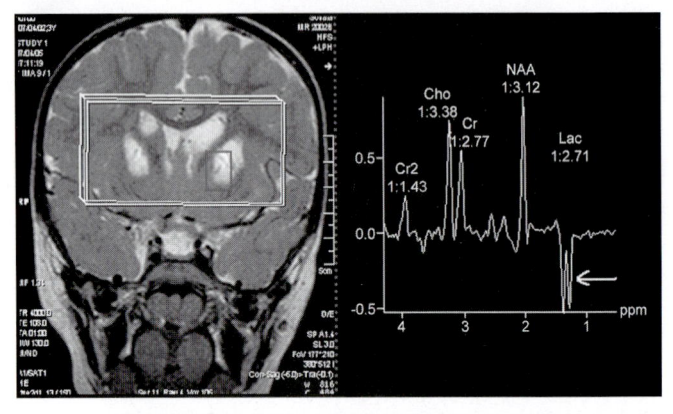

Fig. 14.9: Lactate peak in metabolic disorder.
Bilateral basal ganglion hyperintensity noted in the this patient of Leighs disease. Note bifid inverted lacate peak at 1.3 ppm (arrow) in this TE135 spectrum

Stroke

NAA and Cr are reduced whereas Cho and lactate are elevated. Extent, severity of ischemia and peripheral penumbra can be defined by CSI.

Closed Head Trauma

In diffuse axonal injury there is decrease in NAA/Cr ratio and absolute concetration of NAA. Outcome correlates with NAA/Cr and NAA values.

Epilepsy

NAA/Cr is reduced in affected lobe. MRS can be used to localise intractable epilepsy.

Multiple Sclerosis

In MS plaques, there is decrease in NAA/Cr and increased Cho/Cr and MI/Cr. Active plaque shows elevated lipid, lactate, Cho/cr ratio and MI. Progression can be monitored by NAA/Cr ratio.

Alzheimer's Dementia

All dementias and aging show reduction in NAA/Cr, NAA and elevation of Cho/Cr ratio. However, Alzheimer's shows increased MI/Cr and absolute MI concentration. Similar findings are seen in dementia associated with Down syndrome.

Hepatic Encephalopathy (HE)

There is reduction in MI and Cho, and elevation of Glx. MRS can detect subclinical HE.

HIV and AIDS

There is steady decline in NAA/Cr in HIV patients. MRS helps to differentiate lymphoma, toxoplasma and PML.

Lymphoma: Elevation of lactate, lipids and choline; reduction of NAA, Cr and MI

Toxoplasma: Elevation of lipids and lactate and reduction of all other metabolites.

PML: Slight elevation of lactate, lipid, elevation of Cho, MI; reduction of NAA, Cr.

Abscess

Abscess can be difficult to differentiate from neoplasm. The changes in MR spectra in abscess include visualisation of amino acid peaks at 0.9 ppm. These amino acids include valine, leucine and isoleucine. There may be peaks representing acetate, pyruvate, lactate succinate, which are end products arising from microorganisms.

CHAPTER 15

Cardiac MRI

INTRODUCTION

Cardiac MRI (CMR) opens a new era into cardiac imaging with the potential to provide virtually all of the information needed to assess heart disease. It gives anatomic and functional diagnosis in acquired and congenital heart disease. It has already become the modality of choice in conditions like ARVD, differentiation of constructive pericarditis from restrictive cardiomyopathy and aortic dissection. It gives precise quantification of ventricular dimension and function. Most exciting application of CMR is assessment of myocardial viability and perfusion.

We will first understand the basics of techniques used, imaging planes and then in short discuss role of CMR in various conditions.

ECG GATING

Image acquisition is done in particular phase of cardiac cycle with every cardiac cycle to avoid image blur and cardiac motion artifacts. Usually R-wave is used to trigger the acquisition after some trigger delay such that data is acquired in diastolic phase (Fig. 15.1).

Peripheral pulse also can be used for gating but it is less effective than ECG gating.

Imaging Sequences

Pulse sequences used for CMR can be broadly divided into dark-blood and bright-blood techniques.

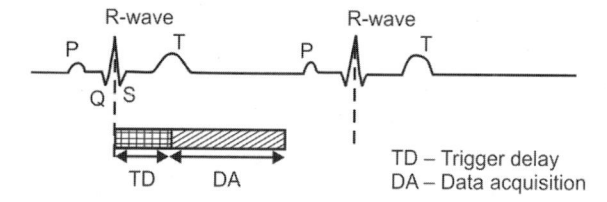

Fig. 15.1: Diagram of ECG gating

Dark-Blood Technique

These are spin-echo sequences that show flowing blood as flow void. It includes conventional spin-echo, breath-hold turbo or fast spin-echo (TSE, FSE), HASTE, and double inversion recovery FSE (Double-IR-FSE).

Bright-Blood Technique

These are gradient-echo (GRE) sequences that show blood bright. GRE sequences used for CMR include turboFLASH and TrueFISP. A motion picture loop through out the various phases of cardiac cycle can be produced with GRE sequences to *get rapid cine imaging*. Cine imaging is useful in functional assessment of ventricles.

As a general rule, imaging should begin with dark-blood sequences to obtain anatomic information and proceed with bright-blood techniques to assess functional abnormalities.

Imaging Planes

Orthogonal planes (axial, sagittal and coronal) used for general chest imaging are not suitable for cardiac imaging because cardiac axes are not parallel to body axes.

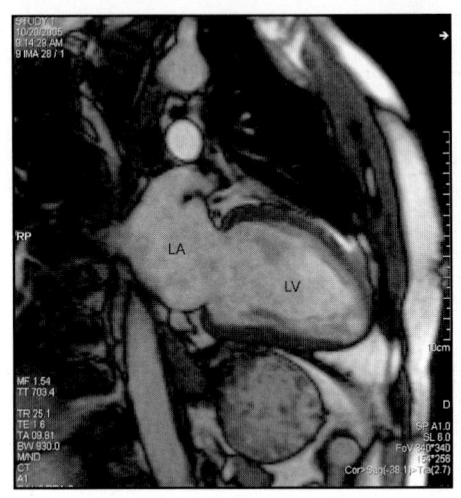

Fig. 15.2: Two chamber view

Imaging starts with axial, sagittal and coronal sections as localizers. Further imaging in planes suitable for cardiac study are based on these images as follows:

1. *Vertical long-axis plane (two-chamber view)* (Fig. 15.2): This is prescribed from an axial image that shows the largest oblique diameter of left ventricle (LV). The two chambers seen are left atrium (LA) and LV. It is useful in assessing left heart structures and mitral valve.
2. *Horizontal long-axis (four-chamber view)* (Fig. 15.3): This is planned from two-chamber view by a line passing through LA, mitral valve and LV. All four chambers, mitral, and tricuspid valves can be assessed together in this view.

Cine GRE images can be obtained in this plane to assess mitral, tricuspid and aortic valve function and RV and LV contraction.

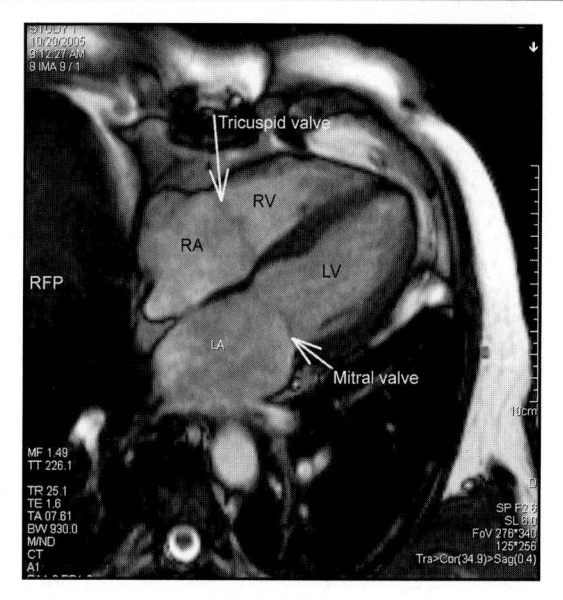

Fig. 15.3: Four-chamber view

3. *Short-axis plane*: Multiple cross-sections are obtained perpendicular to LV long axis as seen on a two-chamber view (Fig. 15.4). These sections are taken from the base to apex of the heart.

   Cine GRE images allow visualization and quantification of systolic myocardial wall thickening. Images in this plane are used to for calculating ventricular volume, mass and ejection fraction by post-processing.

4. *Five-chamber view*: This view is obtained parallel to the line passing through the LV apex and aortic outflow tract on coronal images. Apart from all four chambers,

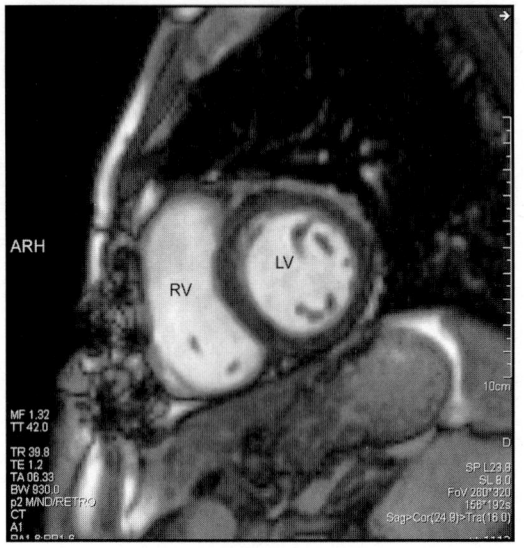

Fig. 15.4: Short-axis view

this view also shows aortic root-the fifth chamber. This plane demonstrates both mitral and aortic valves.
5. *RVOT*: Plane passing through RV outflow tract.

Role of CMR

Congenital Heart Disease (CHD)

CMR is useful in understanding complex anatomy in CHD and gives information not obtained by echocardiography. CMR not only detects ASD, VSD with high sensitivity and specificity but also calculates shunt size with phase-velocity mapping. Using imaging planes aligned with cardiac

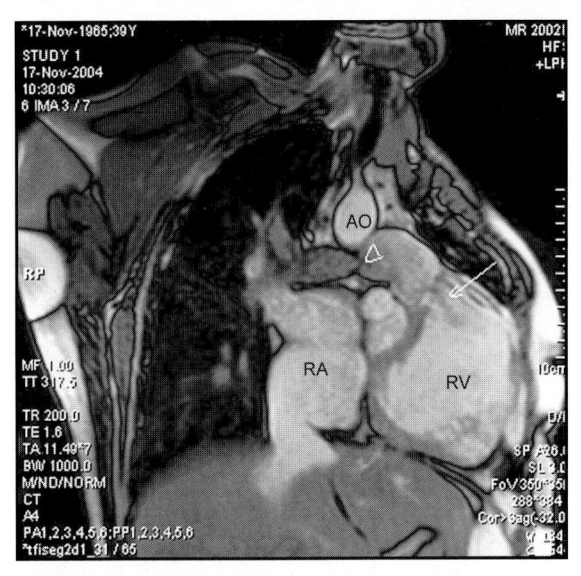

Fig. 15.5: Congenital heart disease. This is a case of tetralogy of Fallot. Note RV hypertrophy, pulmonary regurgitation (arrow) and right pulmonary stenosis (arrowhead)

chambers anatomic details of conditions like transposition of great arteries, truncus arteriosus, double outlet left ventricle and other complex cardiac diseases can be obtained. CMR is also useful for the diagnosis of anomalies of systemic venous and arterial systems (Fig. 15.5). With various treatment options available for congenital heart diseases, survival has improved. CMR plays important role in evaluating complex surgical shunts and baffles with their size as well as function.

226 MRI MADE EASY (FOR BEGINNERS)

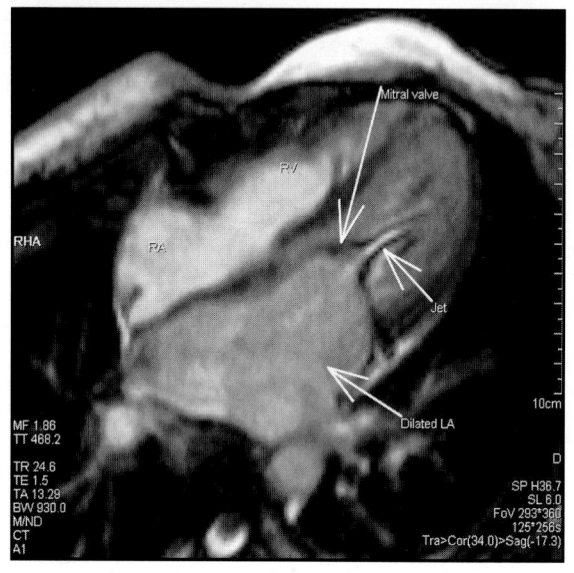

Fig. 15.6: Mitral stenosis

Valvular Heart Disease

CMR can demonstrate the presence and quantify the severity of valvular heart disease. Valvular stenosis or regurgitation appears as dark jet into bright blood containing chambers (Fig. 15.6). The duration or extent of the signal void (jet) on MR images correlates with the severity of the aortic stenosis and total area of signal loss correlates with severity of mitral regurgitation. Direct measurement of the jet velocity can be done using phase contrast technique for assessment of severity and quantification. Cine GRE sequence is useful for leaflets motion assessment.

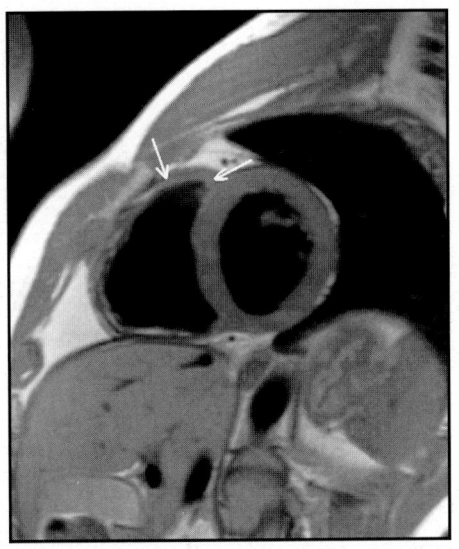

Fig. 15.7: Arrhythmogenic right ventricular dysplasia (ARVD). Short axis view T1-w image shows high density fat in the RV wall (arrow)

Cardiomyopathies

ARVD (arrhythmogenic right ventricular dysplasia) is characterized by fatty or fibrous infiltration (Fig. 15.7) with thinning or thickening of wall and wall motion abnormality of RV free wall. These changes are responsible for ventricular arrhythmias and are one of the causes of sudden cardiac death in young patients. MRI, with its ability to give excellent soft tissue contrast, is the modality of choice for diagnosis of ARVD. Fat in the RV free wall is identified on T1-weighted images. Other findings include thinning of wall, enlargement and dilatation of RV, areas of dyskinesias, focal bulging of free wall during systole, decreased ejection fraction and impaired ventricular filling during diastole.

Hypertrophic cardiomyopathy—Diagnosis is usually made by echocardiography. CMR is useful in the diagnosis of variant confined to the apex and RV involvement. Cine GRE sequences demonstrate the degree and extension of LV hypertrophy. Associated degree of LV outflow tract obstruction and mitral regurgitation can also be assessed by CMR.

Restrictive cardiomyopathy versus constrictive pericarditis—This is a clinical dilemma as both the conditions have same clinical presentation. Differentiation is important because constrictive pericarditis can be treated surgically by stripping the pericardium. CMR reliably differentiates constrictive pericarditis (Fig. 15.8) from restrictive cardiomyopathy by presence of pericardial thickness more than 4 mm. Dark signal void can also be seen suggestive of calcifications. Restrictive cardiomyopathy will have normal pericardium with thickened ventricular walls. It also shows associated complications like mitral regurgitation. Other associated findings seen in both conditions include dilated IVC/SVC, hepatic veins, RA. Causes of restrictive cardiomyopathy include sarcoidosis, amyloidosis, haemochromatosis, scleroderma, storage disorder and idiopathic. Causes of constrictive pericarditis include infective, connective tissue disorders, neoplasm, renal failure, post cardiac surgery and radiotherapy.

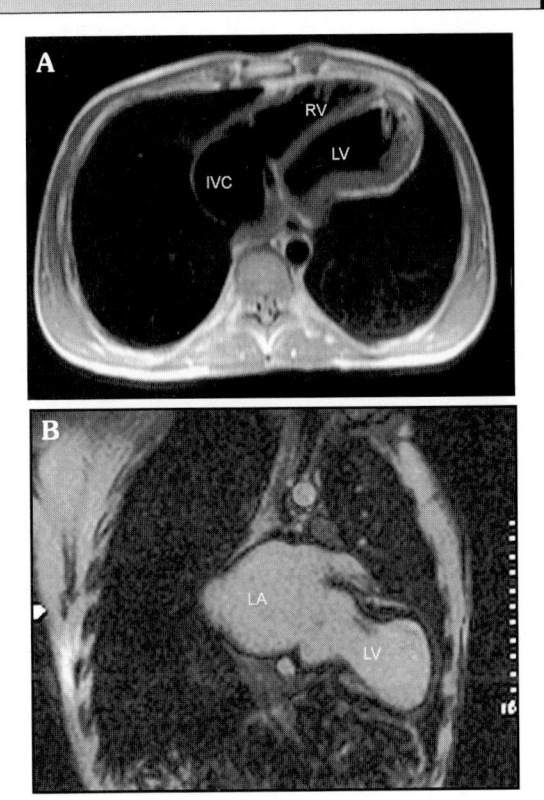

Fig. 15.8: Constrictive pericarditis. HASTE axial image (A) and two chamber view (B). Note small ventricular cavities, dilated IVC and LA. Also seen is thick pericardium at the LV apex

Hemochromatosis—Myocardial iron deposition in transfusion dependant conditions like thalassemia major can be quantified by $T2^*$-weighted sequence. CMR is used to monitor these patients and to assess response to the chelating agents.

Ventricular Function

CMR is reported to be more accurate than 2D echocardiography in functional assessment of the heart. CMR can measure ventricular ejection fraction, end-diastolic and end-systolic volumes. Usually, these measurements are done on short axis images using software. Sequence used is trueFISP that has good contrast between blood pool and myocardium.

Coronary Artery Assessment

CMR still not good for the visualization of distal coronary arteries and branches. Its present role include assessment of anomalous coronary arteries, aneurysm and bypass graft patency. Sequences used are standard GRE with or without contrast injection. TrueFISP is the excellent technique of all.

Myocardial Perfusion and Viability

Myocardial perfusion study—Gadolinium is injected intravenously as tight bolus during pharmacologic stress. Pharmacologic stress is achieved by slow IV injection of adenosine 140 microgram per kg body weight. Sequence usually used is T1-weighted turboFLASH with high temporal resolution. Low signal areas of underperfusion correspond to regions of ischemia or infarct.

Myocardial viability—The imaging sequence for assessment of viability is run after 10-15 minutes of gadolinium injection. Sequences used are IR turboFLASH or trueFISP.

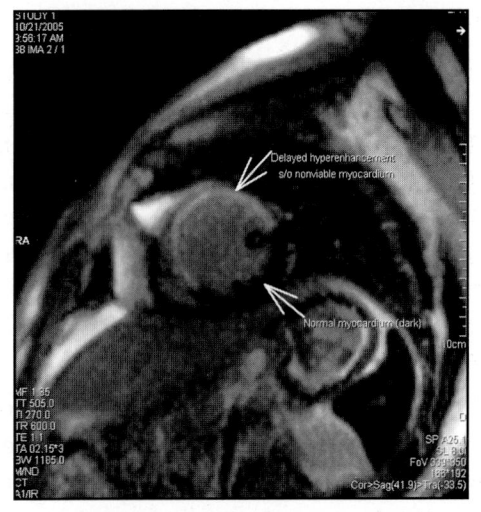

Fig. 15.9: Viability short axis view

Infarcted area on viability imaging shows enhancement or bright signal. 'Bright is dead' on viability imaging (Fig. 15.9). Selection of proper IR pulse (TI-inversion time) is important to suppress signals from normal myocardium.

MR viability answers very important question- whether the patient will benefit from revascularization procedure like angioplasty, bypass or not. It shows the extent and severity of non-viable myocardium. Recent studies have shown that myocardial viability determined by CMR is superior to PET.

Cardiac and Pericardial Masses

CMR is an accurate means to evaluate cardiac and pericardial masses (Figs 15.10A and B). Gadolinium

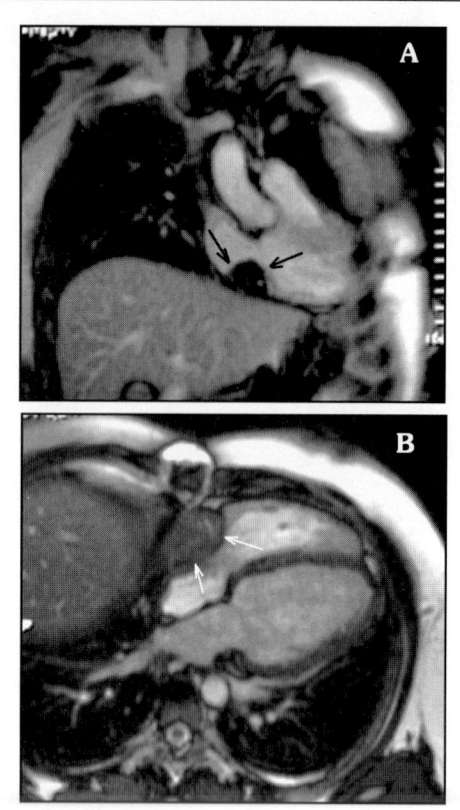

Figs 15.10A and B: Cardiac mass. Coronal (A) and four chamber view (B) image shows mass in RA arrows

enhancement differentiates thrombus from mass, which is the most common filling defect in cardiac chamber. Most of the cardiac neoplasms are secondary or metastatic. Primary cardiac tumors are rare and 80% are benign.

Pericardial Disease

Pericardium can be visualised with spin echo or GRE images. Normal pericardium is seen on spin echo images as a line of low signal intensity located between the high signals of pericardial and epicardial fat. Normal thickness is 1-2 mm; more than 4 mm is thickening.

CHAPTER 16

MRCP

INTRODUCTION

Magnetic Resonance Cholangiopancreatography has got a widespread clinical acceptance and has almost replaced diagnostic ERCP. MRCP visualizes biliary and pancreatic tree non-invasively without use of any contrast injection or radiation. MRCP and ERCP are compared in Table 16.1.

Table 16.1: Comparison of MRCP and ERCP

	MRCP	ERCP
1.	Non-invasive, radiation-free	Involves contrast injection and radiation
2.	MRCP produces images of duct in its natural physiological state	In ERCP ducts are distended with contrast
3.	MRCP can be combined with conventional MR imaging to evaluate extraductal disease	Extraductal pathology or structures can not be assessed by ERCP
4.	Ducts beyond obstruction can be visualized	Contrast may not pass beyond the obstruction. Hence proximal ducts may not seen
5.	MRCP can be performed in post surgical patients in which biliary-enteric anastomosis is performed.	It may not be possible technically to perform ERCP in such patiets.
6.	Non-operator dependant	Operator dependant
7.	MRCP is useful in patients after incomplete or unsuccessful ERCP	Upto 10% technical failures are reported in ERCP
8.	Safe	ERCP involves morbidity and mortality. Complications include pancreatitis, haemorrhage, perforation, sepsis.

Contd...

	MRCP	ERCP
9.	Major limitation of MRCP is its therapeutic incapability	Therapeutic options like sphincterotomy, endoscopic lithotomy, brush cytology, collection of pancreatic juice, stricture dilatation, stent placement and biopsy are possible with ERCP.
10.	Second limitation of MRCP is its less spatial resolution than ERCP.	Higher spatial resolution achievable with ERCP may be important in precise delineation of pancreatic side branches. This is of significance with availability of newer less invasive pancreatic surgeries-segmental pancreatic resection, cyst enucleation.

MRCP TECHNIQUE

Preparation: patient should be empty stomach for 8-12 hours to avoid any fluid in GI tract specially in stomach. If fluid is present in stomach, it can be suppressed by barium or blue-berry juice.

MRCP includes heavily T2-weighted sequences that show stationary or slow-moving fluid, such as bile, as high signal intensity. A number of techniques have been employed to achieve heavy T2-weighting, however, two techniques commonly used include RARE and HASTE.

RARE: Rapid Acquisition with Relaxation Enhancement

RARE is nothing but fast spin echo (FSE) or Turbo spin echo (TSE) sequence in which 90 degree pulse is followed by a train of 180 degree pulses. RARE is a single shot technique acquired as thick slab of 3-7 centimeter with acquisition time of 2-3 seconds. RARE uses long TE in the range of 900ms so that fluid that has long T2 shows bright signal. Signal from background soft tissues, which have short T2, is decayed by the time acquisition done at TE of 900ms. Hence there is no background tissue or source images in RARE. RARE can be acquired as 3D acquisition, which is then postprocessed with MIP.

RARE is also acquired as thin slice acquisition for small intraductal calculi or other filling defects. In this thin slice acquisition TE is in the range of 80-100ms hence background soft tissue are visualised and periductal pathology can be assessed.

HASTE: Half Fourier Single Shot Turbo Spin Echo

HASTE is FSE or TSE acquired as single shot in which only half of k-space is filled. TE used in HASTE is in the range of 80-100 ms so background tissues are not suppressed. Post processing in the form of MIP is needed to get cholangiopancreatogram.

MRCP should also include, depending on the case, other MR sequences to evaluate extraductal structures and pathologies.

CLINICAL APPLICATIONS OF MRCP

Cystic Diseases of the Bile Duct

MRCP is as effective as ERCP in evaluating choledochal cyst, choledochocele and Caroli's disease (Fig. 16.1).

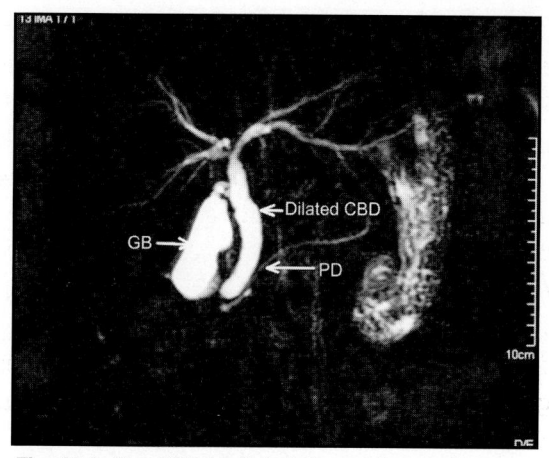

Fig. 16.1: The CBD is dilated, the confluence is normal and there is no IHBR dilatation. These findings are suggestive of choledochal cyst

Congenital Anomalies

Pancreatic divisum—MRCP is superior to ERCP in detecting pancreatic divisum (Fig. 16.2). Congenital variations like low cystic duct insertion, medial cystic duct insertion, parallel course of the cystic and hepatic duct, aberrant right hepatic duct are visualised on MRCP. Detection of these variations is important to avoid complicatons during cholecystectomy specially laproscopic.

Biliary atresia—MRCP can non-invasively establish the diagnosis of biliary atresia.

Choledocholithiasis

Accurate diagnosis of stones in CBD is important before cholecystectomy. MRCP is an excellent method to detect

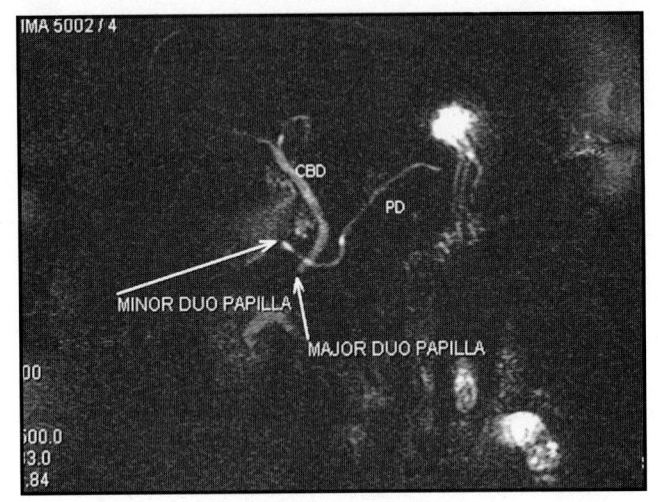

Fig. 16.2: Pancreatic divisum

these stones, comparable to ERCP and superior to other modalities like USG and CT (Figs 16.3 and 16.4).

Primary Sclerosing Cholangitis

It is characterized by multiple irregular strictures and saccular dilatations of the intrahepatic and extrahepatic bile ducts producing beaded appearance. MRCP is useful in the diagnosis and follow up of primary sclerosing cholangitis. ERCP may result in progression of cholestasis and may not show ducts proximal to severe stenosis.

Postsurgical Complications

Postsurgical complications like benign strictures, retained stones, biliary leak, biliary fistula are effectively evaluated with MRCP (Fig. 16.5).

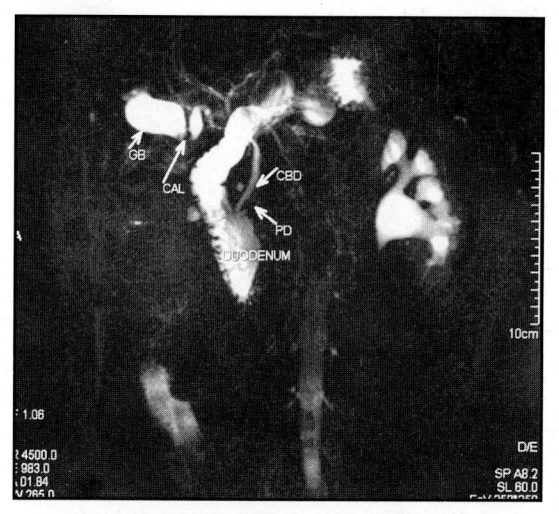

Fig. 16.3: Calculus in the GB

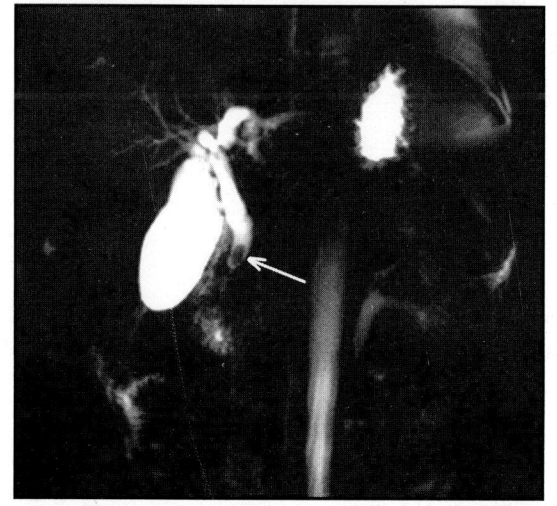

Fig. 16.4: Calculus in the CBD (arrow) with proximal dilatation

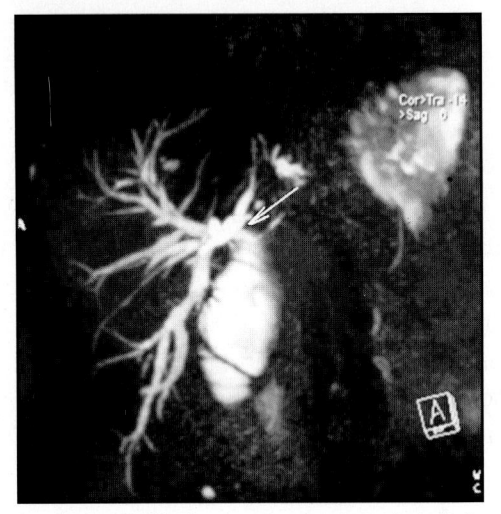

Fig. 16.5: MRCP shows normal patent choledocho-jejunal anastomosis

Chronic Pancreatitis

Chronic pancreatitis is characterized by pancreatic duct dilatation, narrowing or stricture and irregularity. Alcoholic chronic pancreatitis is usually heterogenous and characterized by side-branch dilatation and ductal calcifications whereas obstructive pancreatitis is more homogenous, lack calcification and is associated more often with main duct dilatation. MRCP is useful for detecting chronic pancreatitis and for identification of a surgically or endoscopically correctable lesion.

Neoplastic Lesions

MRCP can show duct proximal to obstruction caused by neoplasms like cholangiocarcinoma and pancreatic head carcinoma. Conventional MR imaging like fat saturated post contrast T1-weighted images should be combined with MRCP for the evaluation of extent and spread of the lesion.

Secretin MRCP (s-MRCP)

Secretin is a hormone that stimulates exocrine pancreatic secretions and distends pancreatic duct. s-MRCP, performed after administration of secretin, is useful for functional imaging and improved anatomic depiction of pancreatic ductal system. It reduces the false-positive depiction of strictures. The main limitation for s-MRCP is the high cost of secretin.

CHAPTER 17

Miscellaneous MR Techniques

fMRI : FUNCTIONAL MRI

fMRI is a non-invasive MR technique to map or localise brain areas which are responsible for particular task. Patient is asked to perform particular activity e.g. finger-thumb apposition and the sequence- usually T2*-weighted EPI, is run. The areas responsible for the activity (e.g. sensory motor cortex) will show increased signals.

Mechanism

fMRI is based on technique called as Blood Oxygen Level-Dependant (BOLD) imaging. DeoxyHb (Deoxyhemoglobin) is much more paramagnetic than OxyHb. Paramagnetic agents cause drop in signal on T2 or T2*-weighted images.

When any brain area is activated by the particular task, blood flow to that area increases (Fig. 17.1). This increase in blood flow is much more than the metabolic demand. This increase in blood supply results into more of oxyHb and less of deoxyHb in that area. This results into increased signals because deoxyHb is reduced, which is responsible for decrease in signal on T2 or T2*-weighted images.

Usual areas mapped and tasks include-
1. Finger tapping /apposition of thumb with fingers for sensory motor cortex activation
2. Light flashing for visual cortex.
3. Sound tones for auditory cortex.

Why do we map brain areas by fMRI?
Apart from ongoing research in understanding brain

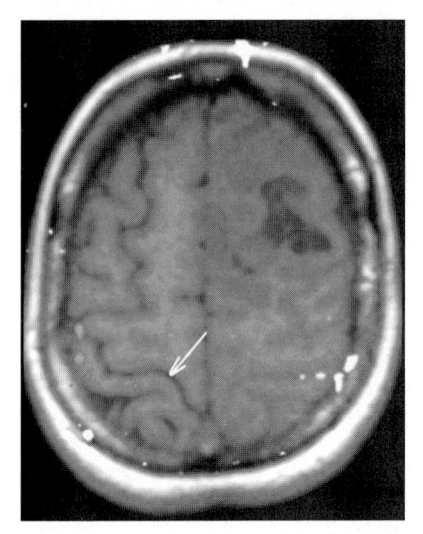

Fig. 17.1: Functional MRI. BOLD image shows an activated red area on finger movement of right hand in the postcentral gyrus (motor cortex). Arrow indicates central sulcus. Patient has a tumor in left frontal lobe

functional areas and understanding psychiatric diseases, fMRI has clinical uses like-

1. Estimation of risk of postoperative deficit, e.g. if the particular functional area is more than 2 cm away from the tumor or lesion to be resected, then patient is less likely to develop postoperative deficit.
2. Determination of hemispheric dominance for language.

CSF FLOW STUDIES

There is continuous to and fro movement of CSF with cardiac cycle. During systole, because of expansion of cerebral hemispheres, there is craniocaudal movement of the CSF from lateral to third to fourth ventricle. During diastole CSF moves cuadocranially. On conventional MR imaging this manifests as flow void in the acqueduct.

CSF flow studies are done by phase contrast method, which is used also for MR angiography and venography. The study is performed with ECG gating that could be prospective or retrospective. It is usually done for acqueduct with acquisitions in-in-plane (along the acqueduct) and through-plane (perpendicular to the acqueduct). At the end of examination what we get is magnitude images (showing anatomy), phase images or CSF flow images (giving information about CSF flow) and data from which acqueductal stroke volume is calculated (Figs 17.2A to D).

On CSF flow images CSF in acqueduct is bright during systole (craniocaudal flow) and dark during diastole (caudocranial flow). Normal acqueductal stroke volume is 42 microliters. Stroke volume more than 42 microlitre is suggestive of hyperdynamic flow.

Clinical Applications of CSF Flow Studies

1. NPH—Normal Pressure Hydrocephalus
   NPH is a condition in elderly patients with clinical triad of dementia, gait disturbances and incontinence of urine. In NPH mean intraventricular pressure is normal (compensated hydrocephalus) but the pulse pressure is increased several times. This pulse pressure pounds against paracentral fibers—corona radiata ('water-hammer pulse') and also causes compression of the

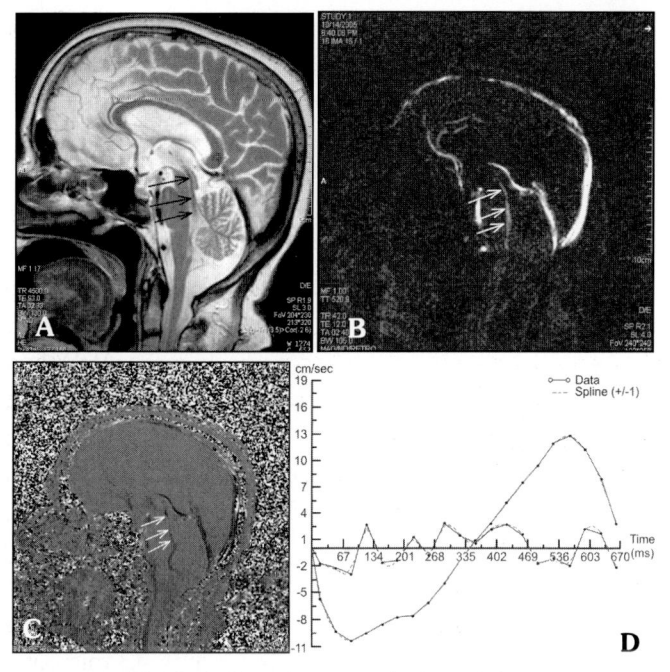

Fig. 17.2: Normal pressure hydrocephalus.
T2-w sagittal image of the brain (A) shows hyperdynamic jet in the aqueduct (arrows). In-plane CSF flow study-Magnitude image (B) and Phase image (C) shows flow in the aqueduct (arrows). The graph of CSF flow plotted against cardiac cycle (D). Note flow below baseline during systole and above baseline during diastole

cortex resulting into symptoms. Conventional MR images show ventricular dilatation out of proportion to the sulcal widening. In NPH there is hyperdynamic flow (increased to and fro motion) that manifests as increased flow void in acqueduct on routine MR images.

If this flow void is extensive, from third ventricle to fourth ventricle through the acqueduct, then there is good response to ventricular shunting, which is treatment for NPH.

Acqueductal stroke volume more than 42 microliter on CSF flow studies has good response to ventricular shunting. Patient with stroke volume less than 42 microliter is less likely to benefit from shunting. Thus MR has diagnostic as well as prognostic value in NPH.

2. Shunt evaluation—Ventricular shunts have stop valve that allows unidirectional flow. So on flow images of the patent shunt signal during systole-diastole will be bright-gray-bright-gray. If shunt is blocked signal in the tube will be gray in both systole and diastole.

   After shunting flow through the acqueduct is reversed (caudocranial during the systole) because of low pressure pathways through the shunt for the CSF that is pushed upwards by cerebellum and choroid plexus in fourth ventricle. So if the flow in acqueduct is normal (i.e. craniocaudal during systole), it is suggestive of shunt block.

3. CSF flow studies are useful in differentiation of arachnoid cyst from mega cisterna magna. Arachnoid cyst will show movement during systole and diastole and will show different flow than surrounding CSF.

MAGNETIZATION TRANSFER IMAGING

MT is a technique which selectively alters tissue contrast on the basis of micromolecular environment. Tissues normally have three pools of hydrogen protons that are responsible for MR signals. These are-

1. Free-water protons
2. Bound or restricted water protons in macromolecules
3. Hydration layer water protons adjacent to macromolecules

In routine imaging protons from free water pool are responsible for most of MR signals in an image because of their long longitudinal relaxation time (T2). Protons from other two pools have very short T2, hence contribute little to MR signal.

Range of resonance frequency or spectral bandwidth of free pool is narrow while restricted pool has wide spectral bandwidth.

Restricted pool can be saturated by applying RF pulse at anywhere its spectral width. Once saturated, protons of restricted pool exchange their magnetisation with protons of free pool via hydration layer protons. This occurs through a process called 'dipolar coupling'. This results into reduction of T2 of restricted pool or macromolecules and reduction in their signal intensity. The increase in image contrast thus achieved is called MT contrast (MTC). Amount of signal loss on MT images reflect amount of macromolecules in given tissue.

MT pulse is applied as off resonant RF pulse to water peak. It is usually applied as presaturation pulse, at +1000 Hz, opposite side of fat saturation pulse (at -220 Hz) (Fig. 17.3).

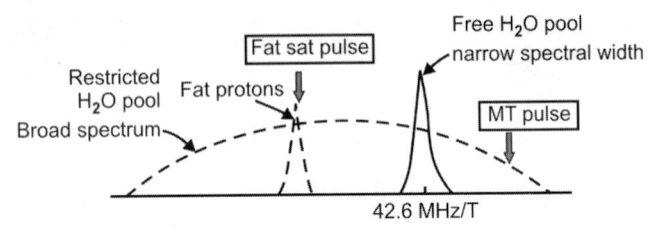

Fig. 17.3: Diagram of magnetization transfer

APPLICATIONS OF MTC

1. Contrast enhanced MRI—MT suppresses background tissue signals while affecting negligibly to enhancing lesion or structure. Thus improves visualization of the lesion (Fig. 17.4).
2. MR angiography—MT suppresses background tissue while preserves signals from blood vessels resulting into improved small vessel visualization.
3. Pathology characterization—apart from increasing conspicuity of enhancing lesion MT is also being studied to characterize lesions into benign and malignant depending on their macromolecular environment and high molecular weight nuclear proteins.

MR MYELOGRAPHY

It is analogous to conventional myelogram but does not involve injection of any contrast or radiation. Basic principle is same as MRCP where heavily T2-weighted sequences are used to visualize static or slow flowing fluid. Sequences used are same as MRCP- HASTE and RARE. MR myelogram forms the part of spine study and takes about 30-40 seconds for acquisition (Fig. 17.5).

MISCELLANEOUS MR TECHNIQUES 253

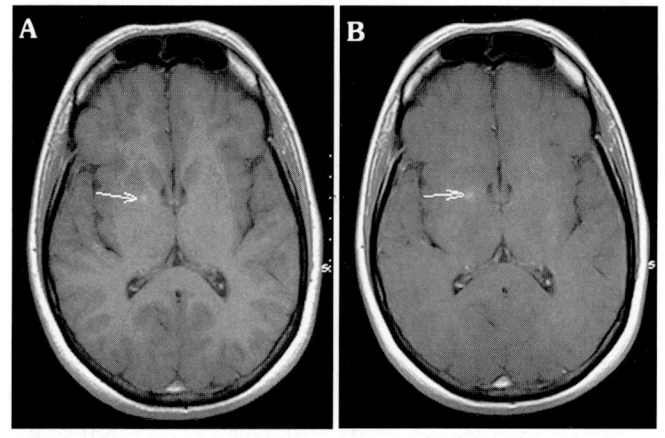

Fig. 17.4: T1-w post-contrast axial image (A) of the brain shows an enhancing lesion in the right globus pallidus (arrow). With magnetization transfer on (B) the conspicuity of the lesion increases (arrow)

MR Urography

As in MRCP and MR myelography, heavily T2-weighted sequences like HASTE and RARE are used for visualization of pelvicalyceal system.

MR urogram can also be performed with IV contrast-Gadolinium. This is specially useful in patients with compromised renal function as Gadolinium is non-nephrotoxic. After injection of IV gadolinium, images are acquired in similar

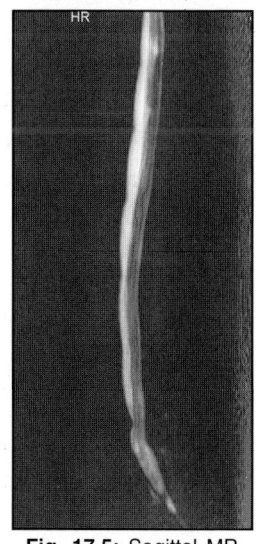

Fig. 17.5: Sagittal MR lumbar myelogram

fashion to IVP at 0, 1, 5, 10, 15, 20 minutes. Sequence used is T1-weighted FLASH, which are post processed with MIP to get images of pelvicalyceal system.

MR Arthrography

MR arthrogram involves passive distension of the joint space and MR imaging for the joint.

Procedure: A solution is injected in the joint space under fluoroscopy guidance. The solution is made up of 0.1 cc of Gadolinium (for contrast in MR images), 2 cc of water soluble iodinated contrast media (for visualization of joint space under fluoroscopy) and 20 cc of normal saline. Patient is imaged within 45 minutes of joint injection with routine sequences.

Indications

1. Recurrent dislocation of the shoulder joint. MR shoulder arthrogram allows visualisation of the glenoid labrum, glenohumeral ligament and rotator cuff in exquisite detail (Fig. 17.6). MR arthrogram shows anteroinferior labral detachment (Bankart's lesion), APLSA (anterior labrum periosteal sleeve avulsion), GLOM (gelnoid labrum ovoid mass) and SLAP (Superior labrum anterior-posterior) lesion in recurrent dislocation.
2. Hip joint.

Stress MRI of Spine

Stress MRI is a new concept in MR imaging of the spine. It is based on the concept that during weight bearing or standing position there is crowding of structures in spinal canal that makes the patient symptomatic. So

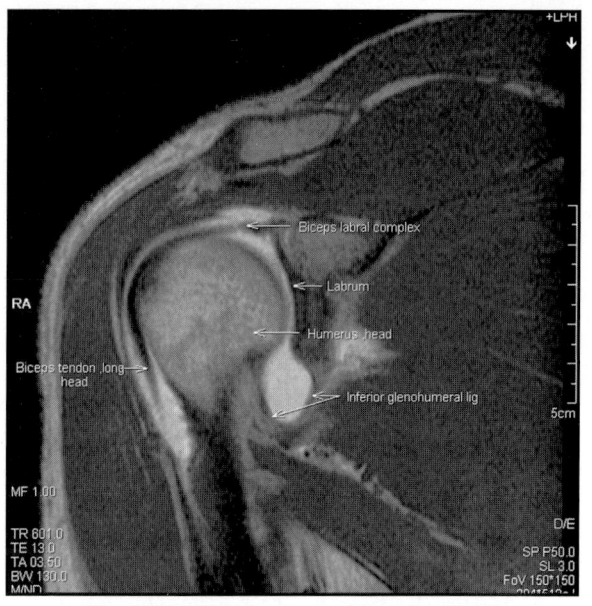

Fig. 17.6: MR arthrogram of the shoulder

imaging the spine in supine position may not depict the actual picture of the pathology.

In stress MRI, standing is simulated in supine position by axial loading. Axial loading is nothing but compression of the body by special equipment which compresses the body by shoulder straps and foot plate. Weight applied is usually 40-50% of patient's body weight. Post-loading scanning should be started after waiting for five minutes.

Scans are acquired pre and post loading and spinal canal area is calculated (Figs 17.7A to D). Stress MRI

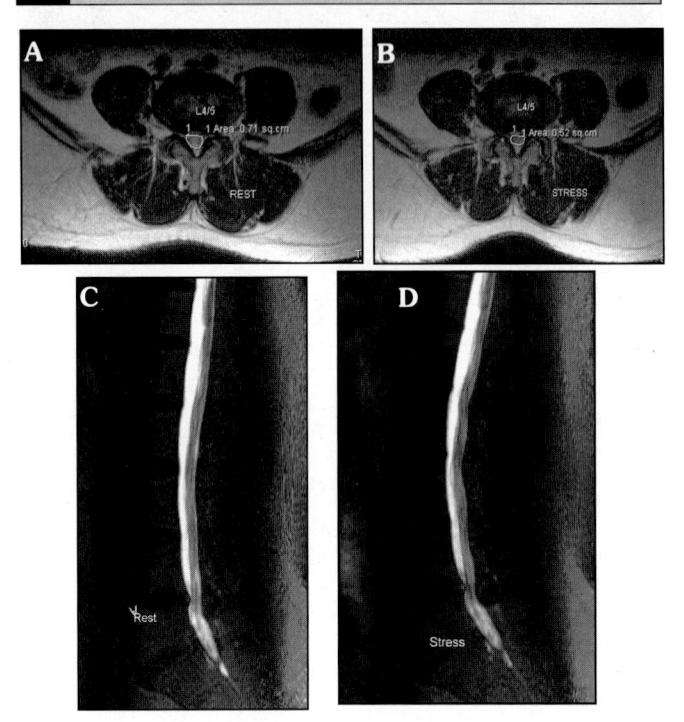

Figs 17.7A to D: Stress MRI of the spine
T2-w axial image of the lumbar spine without stress (A) shows lumbar canal area of 0.71 sq cm, which reduces to 0.52 sq cm on stress (B). Note the effect on MR myelogram as well. (C) at rest. (D) on stress

is presently done only for lumbo-sacral spine. Clinical implications of stress MRI are not yet fully studied. Contraindications include severe osteoporosis, trauma/ fracture, tumor, severe cardiopulmonary compromise, and standard contraindications for MR examination.

Index

A

Acoustic noise 107
ADC map 174
Aliasing 91
Anisotrophic diffusion 172
Arterial spin labeling 192
ARVD 227

B

Bandwidth 23
Black blood imaging 160
BOLD 246
Bright blood imaging 160
b-value 173

C

Cardiomyopathy 228
CBF 185
Chemical shift 92-95, 199
Choline 209
CISS 74
Coherent TM 57
Contraindications 114
Creatine 208
Cross talk 102
CSF flow study 247
CSI 201

D

DESS 84
Diffusion tensor 179
Dipole-dipole interaction 117
Double echo 46

E

Echo train length 48
Electromagnet 28
EPI 60

F

FLAIR 51-53, 70
FLASH 57, 68
Flip angle 22
Four chamber view 222

G

Gadolinium 118
Ghosts 88
Gibbs artifact 97
GMR 163
Gradient echo 54
Gradients 9, 35

H

HASTE 81, 238

I

Inversion recovery 49
ISIS 201
Isotrophic diffusion 172

K

K2 map 186
Key hole imaging 62
k-space 42

L

Larmor frequency 5
Longitudinal magnetization 6
Longitudinal relaxation 14
LOTA 63

M

Magnetic susceptibility 97
Magnetization transfer 250
Magnetism 26
Matrix 22
Mean curve 125
MEDIC 85
MPRAGE 75
MR arthrography 254
MR myelography 252
MR urography 253

N

NAA 207
NPH 248

P

PACE 63
Pacemaker and MR 112
Parallel acquisition 62
Permanent magnet 28
Phase contrast 166
Precautions in MR 113
Precession 4
Pregnancy and MR 109
PRESS 201
Proton density 19

Q

Quench 32

R

Ramping 32
RARE 58, 237
rCBV 185
Resonance 8
RF coils 36
ROPE 63, 90

S

SAR 107
Saturation band 64
Secretin-MRCP 243
Shading artifact 101
Shielding 34
Shimming 33
Signal 8
Spin echo 44
Spoiled TM 57
SSFP 57
Steady state 55
STEAM 59, 201
STIR 51-52, 76
Straight line artifact 99
Stress MRI 254
Superconducting magnet 30

T

T1 16
T2 16
T2 shine through 174
T2* 55
TE 17, 48
Tensor diffusion 179
Tesla 27
TI 49
Time of flight 162
Tissue suppression 50
TONE 64

TR 17, 48
Transverse magnetization 7
Transverse relaxation 15
True FISP 80
Truncation artifact 96
Turbo factor 48
Turbo spin echo 47
Two chamber view 222

V
Viability 230
VIBE 85

Z
Zipper artifact 100